30 day Paleo weight loss plan

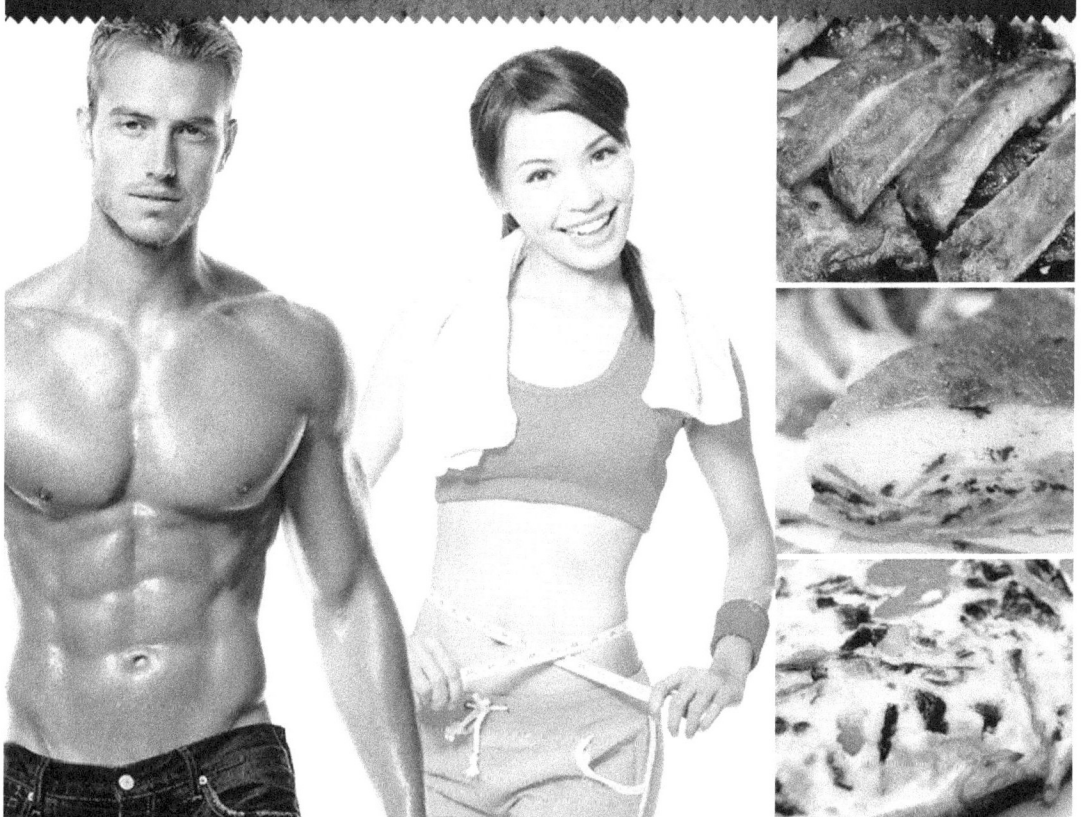

The solution and the science to lose fat fast and live healthy long term

Ceps Weston Domingo

Thanks for purchasing! It means a lot that you would put faith in me and I want to give something back. I give FREE information about fat loss, training, nutrition and recipes on my website: Paindoesnthurt.com

I want the best for you and all I need you to do is go to the website and subscribe where it says Let's do it!

I know you will be happy with the results if you apply the information here and put as much effort as I have presenting this information to you. If you would like to tell me about your results feel free to via my website!

Enjoy the book and do the work! Let's do it!

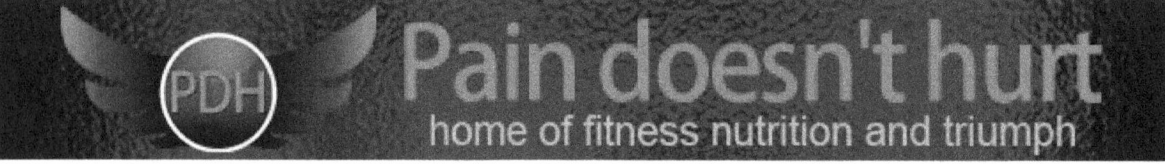

30 day Paleo weight loss plan: The solution and the science to lose fat fast and live healthy long term

By Ceps Weston Domingo

© Copyright 2014 Ceps Weston Domingo

This publication is designed to provide accurate and authoritative information in regard to the subject matter covered. It is sold the understanding that the publisher is not engaged in rendering legal, accounting, or other professional services. If legal advice or other expert assistance is required, the services of a competent professional person should be sought.

First Published, 2014

Printed in the United States of America

Medical Disclaimer

The contents of this book are presented for information purposes only and are not intended as medical advice, nor to replace the advice of a physician or other health care professional. Anyone wishing to embark on any dietary, drug, exercise or lifestyle change for the purpose of preventing or treating a disease or health condition should first consult with, and seek clearance and guidance from, a competent health care professional. The decision to utilize any information in this book is ultimately at the sole discretion of the reader, who assumes full responsibility for any and all consequences arising from such a decision. The author and publisher shall remain free of any fault, liability or responsibility for any loss or harm, whether real or perceived, resulting from use of information in this book.

Table of Contents

Prologue

"You found me beautiful once."

"Honey you got real ugly"

Ash Williams – Army of the dead 1992

With a murderous thud and a battle cry that was as ferocious as the beast he had conquered, there, he stood alone. Victorious. His dense and muscular physique heavy from the battle, his heart racing, the thought was slowly surfacing that he had survived. The massive beast that he had slain was now to be his nourishment, and sustenance for his family. At least for the time being…

His body so strong, so vibrant, he had walked for miles dragging this creature, and so happy he was when he was welcomed by the smiles and cheers when he had reached his small tribe and family. For they all would celebrate his victory with a feast that would nourish men, women and child. Robust and strong they all were for the physical life they had lived. Healthy and alive they all were for the food that nourished them…

Fast forward a few thousand years………

His body was heavy. His lungs were burning. The sweat was pouring and the will was tested.

A "champion" arose out of bed at 5:00AM. He opened the door to the nice cold greeting of the winter air and told himself that he "would go out there and tackle the task at hand". What was this task? It was to run 5 kilometers. The adrenaline flowed, it was him against nature, just him and the cold hard pavement he had to transverse. Right from the start he would give it all that he had got and go till he could not do any more or until the distance was covered.

He felt on top of the world. It was him against all odds. Nothing was going to stop him. Then it happened. He literally fell to the ground and regurgitated last night's takeaway and probably some of that ice cream he had eaten that same day. Maybe the homemade pizza he had eaten for lunch too?

He had looked at his stop watch only to see "2 minutes 30 seconds" and as he had seen that, he then recollected what he had done since he had got out of bed at 5:00AM. He didn't even cover a quarter. Half way? It was a dream. He didn't complete the task. He went until he could do no more but his best was only a mere couple of minutes? Angrily and disgusted in himself he walked his broken body and spirit back home.

Fast forward to now 2013…

What happened to that kid? He had changed. People now talked to him with respect, he had a new found confidence to be comfortable in his own skin, and he was now more vibrant and livelier than ever. He also knew he was a warrior, a primitive one at that. Now, he has reclaimed what he knows so to be true from eons ago as his ancestors have gave him the gift of being one of the many that are carrying their proud heritage in him. He eats to nourish himself. He trains to strengthen and discipline. His outside appearance reflects his drive and determination inside. His whole entire lifestyle shows in his body that he has earned his right to be healthy and strong.

Who was this kid? This kid was me. Ceps Weston Domingo.

It took many years to try things out and get to where I wanted my body to be, and before the word and diet paleo even had came to be in the fitness community what it is now I have been living this life style for years. From that moment I decided I didn't like the Hawaiian homemade pizza being forcefully removed from my body, I took it upon myself to eliminate the junk and nourish my body with only the best foods. Since then I have become qualified in fitness, researched endlessly, trained a lot of other people, and most of all, gave them results.

This book is made for everyone who is serious about losing the fat and attaining the body that they want to have and to be comfortable in their own skin.

Walking through the doors you can expect to learn only the tried and true methods and why they work. You can also expect to learn what foods to eat, what foods to avoid, why you should, and even a list of harmful ingredients that are in your food. Though there will be some technical jargon I promise it is limited since I'm sure you wouldn't want to learn a new language from mars. Or if we're being funny, Uranus, but apparently that isn't a planet anymore.

Walking further down the room you'll be able to see how to put all what you have learned together in order to lose fat and to be healthy at the same time. This book is something you can use, not just something you read.

Right before you enter the doors I am already giving you the weapons you need to get into the mindset to accomplish the goal of getting that body you want. Because ultimately that is why I wrote this book. So you can get results!

You'll find all throughout this book it is all practical information with no useless filler involved. This is the accumulation of all the hard work I have put in for myself, for clients I have trained and all the study and qualifications I have obtained. Want more practical anus kicking? I added at the end of every chapter cliff notes so you can better understand or you can skip right ahead to see what you can expect and even implement some of the things that is in the chapter!

So walk tall with me and let me show you the way. With all that said let's ROCK!

Chapter one: Answers to the question WHY?

"The genius of our ruling class is that it has kept a majority of the people from ever questioning the inequity of a system where most people drudge along, paying heavy taxes for which they get nothing in return" – Gore Vidal

Why should you even attempt to lose the fat in the first place?

In order to do something it makes sense to start with why we should do it. So let's start with first answering the question as to why you should start on this journey towards being that beautiful and vibrant (and if you're the naughty type) luscious minx at the beach.

If I had to say what are three out of the many health risks of having excess fat it would be the following in no particular order:

Firstly obesity and rapid weight gain is one cause of having type 2 diabetes. "The magnitude and the rate of weight gain were also independently associated with diabetic retinopathy. These results quantitative the increased risk associated with magnitude and rate of weight gain"(1). Obesity is something that plagues a lot of people today. If you are overweight and still don't have it, now is the time to do something about it before you keep gaining weight and you do have it. Diabetes can affect your life in such a major way.

Secondly being overweight tends to have an affect on the duration of sleep and that even goes for children! How much? According to a study from Brazil (and don't mind the grammar) "Children with overweight had, on average, 0.39 hours less sleep than those with normal weight"(2). Studies have shown that sleep is "positively correlated with resting energy expenditure adjusted by fat free mass"(3). What this means is that the less fat you have on your body (and muscle is part of your weight so leaving this out), the less energy your body requires to even keep you alive during rest (your resting energy expenditure), and that is correlated to how well you sleep!

The third one is your heart. In my opinion this is the most important. Your heart always beats, even when you sleep. As soon as it stops beating you die. Doesn't it make sense to take care of it? A long term study on the effects of weight gain in 6903 men had showed by the 34.3 years follow up that **"1253 (18.2%) men were discharged from hospital with a principal or secondary diagnosis of Atrial fibrillation".** Not only that but "As expected, cardiovascular risk factor profile deteriorated with increasing weight gain" (4).

These are all just to do with health. How much more are the benefits of losing the unwanted fat for your self-image, confidence and happiness? Reality is, you can truly be the greatest and most kind human being inside but you will get be much more respected if you were 1/4th as kind and you had a body that was a picture of health. Now note this doesn't give you permission to act like a complete anus-hole once you do succeed at your goals!

Where there's a will there's a way combine that with knowledge and you have success: What results to expect

There might be a lot of diets you have tried or even read about. At every turn in the fitness industry it seems like there's always something new popping up and as if there were some miracle. Well I'm here to tell you there isn't any secret at all. You bring the effort and work I'll provide you with the knowledge. Do this and you'll surely have the results you are after.

What exactly is this knowledge I'm about to impart? Is it something mystical or majestic? Unfortunately ladies, unicorns don't exist, and unfortunately guys, there are no 3-boobied girls in real life like from total recall. So basically no the knowledge I will impart isn't mystical or majestic either. However I will say that the results over-time IS seemingly majestic and mystical.

What kind of results can you expect? If you do things right you should be able to lose a pound to two pounds of consistent fat gain a week. That in itself is the miracle! Imagine this scenario. You wanted to lose 10 pounds. The first 30 days you lose 8. So by the 5th week you'd have reach 10 pounds if you kept consistent and thus reaching your goal! If you're like me and you like to prepare for the worst, and say you lost only 1 pound a week. Then I'll tell you in one year you'd lose 52 pounds of fat total if you kept consistent and that is A LOT of fat to lose.

Putting numbers aside you'll also receive the benefit of having a better body with this approach. The reason is simple. If you lost your muscle (and yes muscle is part of your weight on your body too) and you stripped out all the fat along with it you wouldn't look very good nor would you be very vibrant or strong.

If you are starting from a weight that deems you as the heavyweight champion of the world there's good news! You WILL lose MORE weight in the beginning due to water and the excess fat. Your body doesn't need or want the excess fat and therefore it is easier to get rid of at the beginning!

As time goes by and you approach the stages where you are very lean then yes it will get harder but this book will help you make the fat loss consistent no matter what stage you are in. Please also keep in mind that the scale, while it is certainly a tool to measure your progress the best ways to measure your progress is the mirror, feeling parts of your body (as in they're becoming less soft as an example) and the good ol' tape measure to see where you are losing the fat.

There is one more important piece knowledge to impart before we move on, and that is how the fat comes off. As a rule the first place you put on the fat is the last place you lose it and the last place you put on the fat is the first place you lose it. This is why people tend to notice you're losing "weight at the face" because that tends to be the last place you put the fat. Of course when you lose fat your whole body has to lose it too. So don't think that "I'm going to have an anorexic face and nice defined arms but I will still have a beer belly".

Why the number 30 is the most important number for

continuous weight loss

So why is 30 the magic number? Why did I pick that number? Is it because I have a fetish for all things 30? **I want you to now go grab a pen and paper or notepad before we continue and do NOT skip this step.**

Thirty is more of a symbol than a number itself. Thirty represents a month. Some months have more than 30 days and some less. But regardless thirty sums up a month. Thirty days is perfect because it makes good use of the months that are short on days and months that are longer in days. You will use this number for your fat loss and your mindset.

A quote from scientists states that "it takes something 23 times to become a habit" and in my opinion it takes something 30 tries to begin to get used to it. After that you can only get better.

What I want to instill to you in this book is habits. I will be the one to pick the habits for you to choose and do as we get through the book in step-by-step fashion. Many diets and plans fail because they either give something too hard or too fast. All I will be asking from you is to do two habits each 30 days and when you do master that habit you stick with it and then conquer the next two habits and so on.

An example of how this will work is let's say you first have to conquer your challenge of giving up on ordering that pizza or that chocolate ice cream Sunday on your pizza mashed mixed with popcorn that you eat every day. So one habit for thirty days is you choose not to eat the junk food and eat healthy for 6 days in the week and only have the one treat the one meal on one of the days of the week. If this is you starting out, this alone will give you MASSIVE results especially if you combine it with exercise. The rest of the basics in the book will FURTHER accelerate your goals. **Be honest, if this is you right now, write down on that paper or notepad that your first habit is to not eat junk and eat healthy 6 days in the week.**

This is a contract with yourself. The best tools that I'm giving you right now is a notebook and a pen. A calendar (and resist the urge to get one of those fireman calendars ladies), or diary will do too. Simply cross out each day you accomplish the habit and you're well on you way to beating those cravings and getting that body you want.

The mind is where it starts. We can't control the weather, we can't control current events but we can control what we put in our mouth, what we do on a daily basis, and train ourselves physically with exercise and mentally by knowledge and instilling habits.

What is Paleo

Paleo is short for Paleolithic and the "paleo diet" is synonymous with other names such as hunter-gatherer diet, stone-age diet, cave-man diet and more. Seeing as I like my hair short and I like to speak English and read I can't go with those other names. If I had to chose a name instead of paleo I would call it…Actually I'd just call it paleo. But anyway let's forget about the word paleo and all its other various name off-shoots. I want to talk about what Paleo really is and what it stands for!

Paleo is all about getting back to the basics and getting rid of the man-made stuff as well as starches (more on this later). It means to cut out all the chemically laden cattle, food, and all the processed meat and products. Everything that is unnatural we don't want. It's simple. Here's an experiment you can try out for yourself right now. Go to the store and check out a few tuna cans and bread. Look at the ingredients in those and you'll probably not be able to formulate an answer as to what they are or even why they're used. Go see any other product or food that's processed in the shelves and you'll have more time trying to explain things! Right now there might even be a few foods you have at home that you aren't aware what you're actually eating until you see the ingredients!

What Paleo really stands for is to nourish our body with only the best so we can be at our best! To get rid of the worst so we never have to experience the ailments at our worst.

What foods are allowed on this paleo plan?

GRASS FED MEATS, WILD FISH, SEAFOOD

Examples include: Bacon, steak, poultry, chicken, lamb, lobster, bison, goat, salmon, shrimp, eggs, snapper, hoki, muscles, pork, duck, halibut, mackerel, tuna, sardines, tilapia, crab, clams, oysters, scallops, crayfish, and prawn.

VEGETABLES

Examples include: Asparagus, broccoli, cauliflower, kale, leek, bok choy, lettuce, cucumber, eggplant, carrots, celery, spinach, cabbage, tomatoes, parsley and avocado. Sweet potato and beets, while starchy, I'm including to eat because they have good nutritional value and are used for some of the recipes inside of this book. I would suggest not going overboard with them and to eat them moderately.

OILS

Coconut oil, macadamia oil, olive oil, grass-fed butter, avocado oil

NUTS

Almonds, brazil nuts, cashews, hazelnuts, pecans, pine nuts, pumpkin seeds, walnuts, macadamia nuts, sunflower seeds, hazelnuts.

FRUITS

Examples include: Apples, bananas, berries of all kinds, mango, plumbs, peaches, grapes, oranges, figs, tangerine, cantaloupe, watermelon, lemon, papaya, pineapple and lime.

FOOD NOT ALLOWED ON PALEO AND WHY

DAIRY

With the exception of grass-fed butter, 90% of the dairy in the store is chemically altered in someway and to top that off have nasty ingredients in them. They just aren't natural! See that margarine on the shelf that has an expiry date of 5-10 years? How exactly does that product last that long? Trans-fat is what! A lot of people don't know what trans-fat even is or even how to look for it! How about the difference between pasteurized and homogenized milk? What is UHT? We will get further in-depth into the ingredients in the nutrition ammunition section. But the main take away is dairy is off-limits for these reasons.

SOFT DRINKS AND ENERGY DRINKS

Soft drinks are rich in sugar and high-fructose corn syrup and a host of many other ingredients such as caffeine and sweeteners. These will easily wreck your health and not to mention make your quest for that body you want hard.

FRUIT JUICES

While fruit is OK to eat and is a useful tool for athletes, fruit juices have high concentrations of fructose and sugar more so than the fruits. To top that all off some of the fruit juices you see in the store do have other ingredients to make them taste better. All this being said, it's definitely a no-no for the fat loss and definitely not good for diabetics in particular. Same could be said with the soft drinks and energy drinks.

GRAINS

Yes grains! Grains are very starchy and almost all grains contain traces of gluten. Excessive intake of gluten can cause gastrointestinal symptoms in people with and even without celiac disease (31). Grains are things such as cereals, oatmeal (more on this later though), pasta, bread etc.

LEGUMES

Legumes also known as beans have what is called lectins. Lecitins allow harmful material to pass freely from the intestines into his bloodstream. Also the outside of the beans are wrapped in phytic acid which would block the absorption of essential nutrients. Beans take a lot of preparation time if you were to eat them and limit the lectins and the phytic acid which it contains. First you would have to soak your beans for 24 hours and then you would have to boil them thoroughly. Having done this you would eliminate the majority of the bad stuff however there will always be traces so it is best to avoid eating them.

PROCESSED MEATS

Nothing like a hot dog to go with a front row seat to a ball game eh? Processed meats are meats such as hot dogs, spam, processed ham, all other processed packaged meats and all low quality meats.

SNACK FOODS

Ah yes. The memories of pastries and the crackers when you are in front of the TV watching movies or playing video games. You will practically never get full from these foods and you will keep eating and eating. These are definitely one of the worst things to have lying around so conveniently around the house. Not only that, but these have an expiration date that lasts for years! Throw them out or give them to that guy you hate that didn't give your lawn mower back or to that girl that rejected you because she thinks it's weird you can make your chest dance to whatever song was on the radio.

ALCOHOL

I can appreciate that almost everyone in the world likes to have a good time with a drink. I'm all for a good time too and can do so without a cold one. Cutting it out completely might not be something you want to do, and I'll say that you can drink on occasion that's fine! Drinking yourself silly every day or drinking yourself silly at anytime in particular is obviously what you want to avoid.

If you were to drink something I would say red wine would be a good choice. It is shown to give a nitric oxide boost and dealcholised red wine can decrease diastolic and systolic blood pressure (5,6). Not only that, but history says that the honeymoon is a viking tradition and to induce more intimate moments during the honey moon the Vikings would consume something called mead. This was a mix of red wine and honey. Nitric oxide helps blood flow through the body. That means the insane pumps at the gym and the pumps downstairs. To the hardcore paleo crowd I do realize that alcohol might not be considered paleo by they hardcore standards and especially not honey mixed with red wine. But I understand people do want to live life and there will be those social occasions and why not recommend something that will at least let them enjoy those occasions while getting some benefit? It'll also help you all to stick to this plan. Besides, I don't like waking up to hate mail in my inbox with 10 reasons why I should insert a steak kebab down my hamster hole because I'm telling you to give up every single thing there is in life.

The science of the benefits of paleo on health

As you can see from the food listed above on what to eat, you'll notice it is all natural food found in nature and nothing man-made. Leaving out all the bad chemicals and ingredients in food and ensuring you are getting a wholesome and balanced meal. What that means is you'll be getting nutrients and vitamins from a broad spectrum and it will fulfill your daily requirements. Eating this way has numerous benefits. The main and interesting ones are the following:

PREVENT CONGESTIVE HEART FAILURE AND LOWER BLOOD PRESSURE

When you cut out the junk food and eat natural, your diet will have lower sodium intake. The French fries and all that ketchup on your hot dog for instance is loaded with sodium! "Dietary sodium intake was significantly associated with an increased risk of CHF incidence in overweight, but not in non overweight, persons. Furthermore, the relative risks were similar when either sodium-calorie ratio or absolute sodium intake was used as the independent variable."(7) Not only that but it may lower blood pressure and help with hypertension(8).

MAKES SURE YOU LOSE THE UNWANTED WEIGHT IN THE LONG RUN

This plan makes you to keep track of things and the benefits of that in long term weight loss are it's a sure thing. A study shows that "Daily self-monitoring of weight, physical activity, and F/V (fruit and vegetable) consumption is a feasible and effective approach for maintaining weight loss for 12 months"(9).

HELPS DIABETICS

This plan takes into account vegetable consumption and it does control carbohydrates to an extent where it is not so damaging but is used as a tool. A study on Japanese patients with type 2 diabetes has shown that they are able to have much better glycemic control if they eat their vegetables before their carbohydrates. (10).

HELPS WITH PEOPLE WHO JUST QUIT SMOKING TO LOSE WEIGHT AND DECREASES RISK OF GLAUCOMA.

While fruit and vegetable intake alone won't help with weight loss it can help with people who just quit smoking. "The largest difference was observed between strata of smoking behavior. The strongest inverse relation was seen in those who stopped smoking during follow-up". It seems that there is relationship of fruit and vegetable intake and the weight loss in non-smokers. (11)

A suspect reason why fruit and vegetable consumption will help with glaucoma namely has to do with increased consumption of vitamins A and C and carotenoids in the fruit and vegetables (it should be worth mentioning that some meats also have high vitamin A). Of course there might be other specific nutrients in them that will help but this is just the theory. Fruits and vegetables contain many good nutrients and vitamins. (12)

HELPS TO BUILD LEAN MUSCLE

The meat choices are filled with the cholesterol needed to build lean muscle even in older populations. A study on older populations has found the following: "We observed a dose-response relationship between dietary cholesterol (from food logs) and gains in lean mass". (13). Cholesterol in food is very important to have as it is what all steroidal hormones in our body descend from. The testosterone hormone being a main important hormone for muscle gain and sexual drive as an example, in other words, cholesterol produces sex hormones in our body.

PROTECTS CELLS AGAINST FREE RADICAL DAMAGE, INCREASES INTELLIGENCE AND IS HIGH IN B VITAMINS

The meat choices are rich in B-Vitamins (namely B-12), creatinine, taurine and carnosine. The creatinine beneficial for our brain function and is even shown to increase intelligence (44), and it is high amounts of carnosine, an amino acid, that is shown to be an antioxidant, heal wounds faster and protect cells from free radical damage.(43)

Why this plan WILL work

Leonardo da Vinci once said "simplicity is the ultimate sophistication". This plan is all about simplicity. Not only that but this plan will teach you everything you need to know: The basics. Every thirty days will improve a new aspect of you in terms of fitness and fat loss, and while it is challenging, it is do-able!

What is the number one thing that I know this plan will work? You! The more effort you put into this program the more you'll get out of it! 30 days and sticking with those habits from here on takes discipline and effort but the results are great. This plan is realistic, and it is backed up with science. Give this 100% and you'll get 100% it's that simple! It all starts with day one! So with the question why out of the way we can now get to know just what these next 30 days entails! Let's begin!

CLIFF NOTES FOR THE CONFUSED AND IMPATIENT

CHAPTER ONE

1.You should lose fat because: It helps with diabetes, helps with sleep, is good for your heart, self-confidence and happiness.

2.Realistic weight loss: If done right you'll lose 1-2 pounds a week. You'll lose it easier in the beginning. There is no unicorns or 3 boobied girls in real life from total recall.

3. Number 30: signifies a month and every day on that month you will instill a habit

4.Foods allowed: Vegetables that aren't root vegetables, oils that aren't vegetable oils, fruits of all kinds, nuts.

5.Foods not allowed: Dairy, soft drinks, energy drinks, fruit juices, grains, legumes, processed meat, snack foods like potato chips, alcohol (more on this later, red wine can be okay).

6.This plan will: Help prevent congestive heart failure, make you lose weight, helps diabetes, helps with glaucoma, builds muscle, protects against free-radical damage and increases intelligence.

CHAPTER TWO: You don't go to war and win without a plan!

"If you fail to plan, you are planning to fail!" – Benjamin Franklin

The outline of the 30-day plan of attack

This is where we will see the outline on what we will do each and every 30 days. Remember that pen and paper or notebook/diary I told you about? This is where this will come in handy! What you'll also need is a camera, a tape-measure, and a weight scale.

DAY 1: Determine your starting point and establish your goals

As soon as you get up in the morning this is where the day begins for the 30! No excuses! What you now want to do is firstly make sure to go to the bathroom or private place take your clothes off and hop on the weight scale for an accurate weight measure (of course you could do it in front of someone but this is war so no hankey-pankey. Maybe later.)

Next you'll want to measure yourself with the tape measure at your waist (at the navel) your hips, your upper legs (where the hamstring and quadriceps meet), chest and finally arms. Measure them in CM.

Finally we want to determine your lean body mass which is your total weight without the fat and water (so just your muscle weight). To do this you can go to a gym and ask for a trainer to take a skin fold test to calculate your body fat or you can take one yourself by something called an accumeasure which is your own skin caliper you can do at the comfort of your own home. I personally would recommend the accumeasure since you can take the measurement yourself at the same location at the same period of time for just the one fee of buying the caliper, rather than getting a different trainer each time to take a measurement for you and being slightly different each time because of the individual measuring you. You can take this test pretty much anytime in the day, and yes wear clothes. If you absolutely cannot do this test or just plain don't want to for whatever reason then it's not the end of the world. We can still try figure out on how to eat based on your weight and even perhaps a good estimate from what your body fat is by guessing in time. If you go down this route you'll need to keep a closer eye on your food intake though.

We will talk about how to calculate the Lean body mass in the nutrition ammunition section but for now just keep the figure of your weight and body-fat percentage.

Now you have your weight and your measurements of your body sorted I want you now to take a picture of yourself front and side. Make sure that these poses that you do will be the same poses you will have the next 30 days. Make sure you can take a picture of your whole body or at least most of it.

Now you have the numbers and the visual proof you now know where your starting point is for these 30 days. The measurements will tell you where you are losing fat and same as the visual photos. Personally I see dramatic results in the photos every 8-12 weeks but everyone is different and believe me if you do eat well and keep active you will see the results!

So with these numbers you now can determine a goal to set to lose for these 30 days along with the habit you will instill upon yourself. Please set a realistic goal too. Don't say lose 100 pounds in 30 days.

As a good example we'll say that I'm 225 pounds. I eat junk every day for all my meals and I live a sedentary lifestyle and don't exercise at all yet am perfectly capable to do so. My habits for these 30 days will be to eat as this book prescribes for 6 days in the week, with the 7th day having only 2 meals where I eat what I want and exercising the best I can 10 minutes everyday however I like. My minimum goal is to lose 5 pounds these 30 days.

Chances are I will lose more fat and on the 7th day I might feel so good I'll only have one meal where it's complete junk.

The reason I like to have you do this every 30 days is so you know how to adjust and keep going. Use it like a compass. This is to make sure you know you are on the right path!

DAY 2: Determine what to eat, how to eat, and how to lose weight

Every first day in the 30 I like to let people relax a little and just re-asses their goals and starting points as well as get started on their next one or two habits. Day 2 is when the planning starts in terms of eating. So here in Day 2 you'll now map out your battle plan with how much to eat and what to eat. Here is where you should bring your calculator out and another piece of paper. This will give you a familiar idea with the foods and what effects they'll have on you and your fat loss. When you get to know your food you have control.

DAY 3-30: It's time to lose fat and chew bubblegum...And you're all out of gum

You now where you are and you now have a plan with how to eat. You have a map and you have a destination. So it's time to get in there and do it! Day 3-30 is all about keeping consistent with your plan and habits and it's all about taking action every day. After the 30 days are over you will repeat the process again. You'll keep doing this until you are happy with the way you are, and when you are, you'll then have new found knowledge of foods and your body so you can readjust this lifestyle to tailor it to you! Before going on with this book I will want to establish the first two habits

---

30-DAY PALEO HABITS ONE AND TWO
CUT OUT THE JUNK AND MOVE THAT TRUNK:

The first habit as already mentioned, is to get you started by first tackling the act of getting rid of all the junk food, all the takeaways and all the sweets. No matter what position you are in right now in terms of frequency of junk eaten during the week I want you to tackle not eating junk for 6 days in the week and with the 7th day where you can relax. But only by having one junk meal! If that's too hard then you're allowed to have two but that's the max!

REASON FOR HABIT: If you cannot have self-control of eating out, and you cannot learn to say "no" every time you are offered something you know isn't good for you, and you cannot learn how to deal with it then no diet plan in the world will help you. Conquer the food and conquer yourself.

The second habit is to start being active by exercising every day at least 10 minutes a day. Exercise however you like. Weights, bodyweight, boxing etc. Put in your best effort for that day. If you feel like you are great, aren't sore, and not stressed then really go for it! If you are sore and miserable then still train, give some effort but go to how your energy levels and how you feel. The point is to get some activity every day.

REASON FOR HABIT: Using your body as well as strengthening it will build the body you want but not only that it WILL help you lose fat too. Again, you can have the best diet there is but you won't be healthy if you don't use your body in some way. I don't know what complications you, the reader, have in terms of training but any type of physical activity used to strengthen you is needed. Of course I don't want to see you die or hurt yourself in any way (even if it involves naked screaming ladies, and a bad ass minotaur) so please get a medical consent for the all clear in whatever it is you decide to do. If you didn't catch that, yes that is a medical disclaimer.

CLIFF NOTES FOR THE CONFUSED AND IMPATIENT

CHAPTER TWO

1. Grab a pen and notebook or paper, weight scale and camera

2. Day 1 of 30: Assessment day. You will find out your lean body mass which is your weight without body fat, take a photo and measure. You can take your body fat paying a fee every time you ask a trainer at a gym to do it for you or pay a one-time fee and measure it yourself at the privacy of your own home with an accumeasure skin fold caliper.

3. Day 2 of 30: Write up your new eating plan

4. Days 3-30: Kick some adipose tissue in it's collective jewels

5. Habit 1: You will not eat any junk or anything unhealthy for 6 days minimum in the week and can only have ONE naughty meal one day in the week. Naughty you.

6. Habit 2: You will be active and exercise 10 minutes every day. No excuses!

CHAPTER THREE: NUTRITION AMMUNITION

"Thoughts are the gun, words are the bullets, deeds are the target, the bulls-eye is

heaven" – Douglas Horton

You now have the reasons to why this plan works and you have a good idea what the dietary foods to be eaten entails! Here we will finally discuss how the nutrition side of the plan works. What this section will give you is the AK-47 (or if you are a doom video game geek the BFG2000) and the Kevlar vest fat proof body armor to survive the shelves and all the other cons in the dietary industry. Here you will learn ingredients to avoid, some considerations if you are a competitive athlete or diabetic, and how to use the food effectively to lose the unwanted fat you have. It all starts with surviving the macro nutrients!

How to survive macro and micro nutrients: A basic understanding on what they are.

You'll often find that building the body you want is just like building a house. Although if you try build a house yourself you'll need to know what does what and how to use the materials along with the right tools. So first we'll have to understand a little basic knowledge on what macro and micro nutrients are. Learning this in turn not only makes you have knowledge to apply to the food you eat but also makes you aware of what type of dietary trends out there are misleading you!

Macro nutrients are the main components needed in the body. These are your Protein, your carbohydrates and your fats. Micro nutrients are the vitamins and minerals that come along with your food. It's really that simple.

What your body is mostly made out of determines what you should focus on having each day

The major common elements making up all human bodies are the following:

96.1% of the major elements making up the body are **Oxygen, Carbon, Hydrogen and Nitrogen.**

3.9% of the major elements making up the body are **calcium, phosphorus, sulfur, sodium, chlorine, magnesium, iodine and iron.**

Trace elements that make up the body (which are less than 0.01%) are **Cobalt, Chromium, Copper, Fluorine, Magnaese, molybdenum, Selenium, Silicon, Tin, Vanadium, zinc**

What this tells us is that we all need clean, fresh air everyday and to be active. Believe it or not that is part of diet. Oxygen is nourishment. Hydrogen is what influences the pH level of body fluids. Water is very important to drink and you should drink plenty to regulate body temperature and for it to help digestion by making the enzymes work properly in your body. And finally nitrogen is needed. Nitrogen is protein and without protein you WILL waste away. Protein is needed for genetic material, bones, and muscles and more.

So what about the rest? Calcium is needed for muscle contraction and neural transmission along with blood clotting, phosphorus is needed to form part of high-energy ATP, Potassium is needed for contraction of nerve impulses and muscle contraction, sulfur is a component of proteins, sodium is important for water balance conduction of nerve impulses and muscle contraction (although we already have enough of it in the body and unless you were training 8 hours per day you wouldn't need it and as said before it is detrimental if you take too much through food).

Magnesium is important for enzyme activity and metabolic reactions, Iodine is needed to make functional thyroid hormones and iron is needed for oxygen transport in the red blood cells.

As you can see from this a solid balanced diet is necessary and these are the things you should really focus on as they are the major components that make up your body.

What to eat to get all these needs simplified

Now that you'll have a fair idea what does what all you need to think about is firstly ensuring you have a protein source at every meal and to drink plenty of water throughout the day. A gallon of water and more for very active people and especially in hot conditions. The more you sweat the more you'll need. 1.5L is a good start for most. Next you'll need a variety of vegetables and fruits, along with including some nuts. That's it really. Meat fruit and veggies with all your meals and ensuring you cook the food in good nutritious oil like the ones mentioned in chapter two.

Meat will cover your nitrogen needs, fruit and veggies will cover your trace elements and some of your lesser major elements. Nuts will cover nitrogen also and the lesser and trace elements and the oil will cover whatever is missing.

PROTEIN SIMPLIFIED

As already mentioned, protein makes up for the nitrogen needs in the body and is a very essential component. Any diet excluding protein to very low values such as under 40g is a very unhealthy diet. **Protein accounts for over 50% of the major components of the body**.

Protein can come in either incomplete or complete forms. The building blocks of protein are amino acids and the total count of amino acids are 20. Incomplete forms of protein and complete forms of protein mean that the building blocks of protein, which are amino acids, are, as the name suggests, not complete of all 20 or are complete of them. Complete proteins come from animals, which means meat, and not from vegetables, fruits and grains alone. You would have to combine the vegetables and grains to form a complete protein or a legume and a grain. An example is pinto beans and rice to form the complete protein. All animal meats, once eaten, contain all you need. Protein contains hydrogen, oxygen and carbon, sometimes sulfur and they contain nitrogen. Protein has 4 calories per gram.

CARBOHYDRATES SIMPLIFIED

Despite what people say, carbohydrates ARE a useful tool and carbohydrates is the preferred fuel of the body. Carbohydrates instantly turn into glucose. All carbohydrates are sugars. They contain hydrogen, oxygen and carbon. Carbohydrates contain 2 hydrogen atoms to one oxygen atom and this is why the word hydrate in the word carbohydrate is used. Carbohydrates are useful for hydrating the muscles. The true meaning of carbohydrate is that it is a hydrated carbon. As you can see it is very useful for athletes and very active people. However it can also be damaging to people such as diabetics and people who are trying to lose weight. There are three types of carbohydrates. They are monosaccharides, disaccharides and polysaccharides. You don't have to remember the names all you have to remember is the types of food that are good to eat which will be explained right now.

The three types of carbohydrates

Monosaccharide means one sugar. These are the simple sugars that people refer to. The most important ones to remember which you get from food are fructose and fructose. Before nerds go crazy on me yes I am aware there is galactose. Fructose is converted into glucose and any other forms of carbohydrates are converted into that too. Fructose is found from fruit. Fructose in very high unnatural dosages ARE bad. But that is only if you seek to go eat say 100 apples a day or to have things that contain high fructose corn syrup. Natural amounts of fruit won't harm you.

Disaccharides are two sugars. The two sugars are glucose-fructose (sucrose), glucose-galactose (lactose) and glucose-glucose (maltose), found in cane sugar, milk and malt sugar respectively. These types of sugars are to be broken down first to monosaccharides before they can be absorbed.

Polysaccharides means many sugars. Starch is the food that accompanies this. This type of carbohydrate is insoluble. This means that it is perfect for gaining weight! If you wanted to gain weight then you would include this choice, but since you want a nice and in shape body then you would do well to avoid it. Starchy food includes things like root vegetables, pasta and bread. Keep in mind also, it's not just necessarily people who want to gain weight that should include this choice but it's the people that train very hard as if it was their full time job that they should. As you can see this is like a last choice. Inactive people should avoid this.

The bottom line with carbohydrates is to imagine you were filling up a tank of petrol for your car. Let's think of the glucose as the fuel. If you were to have too many you'd spill over the petrol and would have to clean it up. If you were to have a reasonable amount of fuel and used it and filled it up when needed then all is well. The types of carbohydrate are the types of fuel. If you are running a high powered car (a pro athlete doing triathlons for instance) then you'd need the high end fuel (polysaccharides). If you were to be healthy, to look great and be healthy but weren't as active like a pro then you would need standard fuel and focus on the other needs of your body (monosaccharides or disaccharides).

Carbohydrates make up 1-2% of all our cell mass and act as the same as those traffic controllers for planes landing down safely for cellular interactions. As you can see they are important and they are very useful. Now you know how to use carbohydrates efficiently there should be no problems!

FATS SIMPLIFIED

Fats are very important for the body. They help provide the building blocks for cell membranes (every cell membrane is comprised of 40% fat), they can be converted to other substances to perform tasks and namely are important to hormones and they can also be used as energy. In fact fat even contributes to 60% of brain function! Did you know phospholipids have an electrical charge and interact with other molecules in your body such as water? That's right! Fats help the electrical signals in your body. When your communication of your nervous system is impaired just think of the dire consequences with even moving in every day life!

Fat is a pretty hot topic and there is much confusion on this so science is needed a little here but as this section does say simplified I will try my best to make it as simplified as possible. This is crucial to know as you need to be fully aware what fats are actually good for you and what fats aren't.

The types of fat in food consumed are: saturated and the unsaturated fats (monounsaturated and polyunsaturated). Saturated fats are the fats that are solid in room temperature such as butter and unsaturated fats are the fats that are liquid. The body can digest the monounsaturated and saturated fat much easier than the polyunsaturated fat.

Trans fat (we will discuss this more on how to find out what it is in the ingredient section) and highly refined vegetable oils are the unhealthy fats you should avoid. The reason is that they are highly unstable and they become rancid as well as oxidized when they come in contact with heat and even oxygen. Think about why the polyunsaturated fat supplements become rancid quite quickly and tend to have very small shelf life. Why is being oxidized a bad thing? The answer is that they contain reactive compounds which I am sure everyone has heard by now called free radicals. Imagine free radicals like murderous psychopaths with no emotion and only have on purpose: To wreck havoc and kill. These free radicals will attack everything in your body from the cell membranes, the red blood cells and even down to your DNA!

When someone says that something causes inflammation from free radicals they are talking about the damage done by these. I'm sure by now you'll figure what consequences this has on a body. For you fit indestructible men it can mean a variety of chronic ailments, and for you beautiful women it can mean accelerated aging and losing your beauty.

Fats are categorized of either short chain (contains 8 or less carbon atoms), medium chains (8 to 14 carbon atoms), long chain (16 or more carbon atoms) and finally very long chain fatty acids (more than 22 carbon atoms). This is important to know because of how each fat is digested. If you are to replace long chain fatty acid type foods such as any of those vegetable oils (soy, safflower etc.), canola oil or margarine as an example with short and medium chained fatty acids such as butter and coconut oil, you would do your body much more benefit and lose weight much better too. It takes enzymes to even attempt to digest the long chained fatty acids, while the short and medium chains much more readily digested. This means that instead of the fats causing harm to your body you can use the fats for more energy.

Not only that but the short and medium chained fats such as coconut oil is shown to have antioxidant properties to fight free radicals (14) and impede fat gain as well as help lose it! I don't often like referencing a study done on rats to humans but a study has shown that when rats where overfed medium chained fatty acids they had significant results to be noteworthy. "After 4 weeks the rats fed the Medium chained triglycerides compared to the Long chained triglyceride diet weighed significantly less and at the end of the experiment the medium chained triglyceride fed rats had 20% reduction in weight gain and possessed fat depots weighing 23% less." (15).

My advice on oils in terms of which is best to use with all the healthy oils I had already listed that were paleo is coconut oil. The reason is not only the fact it is tasty to cook with and can be used with many recipes but it has an array of benefits such as helping diabetics in regulating blood sugar (of course fat and coconut oil alone isn't the primary cause of regulating blood sugar, if you have a balanced meal with protein that alone is a big reason to help carbohydrates digest slowly), has vitamin E for all you ladies that want good skin and silky hair (think of all the vitamin E and coconut health and skin products on the shelves), has immediate energy and provides antioxidants (it is a medium chained fatty acid) and is a natural antioxidant which means it can help with the immune system and help the body heal and repair (16).

What about the essential fatty acids (EFA'S)?

The essential fatty acids are the omega 3's and omega 6's. They are the monounsaturated and polyunsaturated fats respectively. Our body does require them since the body cannot make any by itself and it must be taken through our daily food. The problem I want to bring up is as discussed, polyunsaturated fats cause the havoc on your body as you can see. Truth is we do not need plenty of these fats. If you intake an excess of the omega 6's (polyunsaturated) you will undoubtedly wreck havoc. So what can you do without wrecking havoc by going into excess? Avoid the oils mentioned and unnatural and all other unnatural products and get the fats from **WHOLE FOODS.** The foods are what I mentioned that are paleo; the nuts, the meats and fish, avocado etc. If you want to take it a step further with the essential fats that your body needs the most eat foods that are high in **EPA and DHA** (notice I said food not oils). Now we have covered everything you need to know in terms of basics of macro nutrients we can now move on to the next step in eating, (that most get confused with) which is meal frequency and timing!

CLIFF NOTES FOR THE CONFUSED AND IMPATIENT

CHAPTER THREE PART ONE

1. Macro nutrients and micro nutrients: Macro nutrients are protein, carbohydrates and fats. Micro nutrients are vitamins and minerals. 96.1% of the major elements making up the body are **Oxygen, Carbon, Hydrogen and Nitrogen.**

3.9% of the major elements making up the body are **calcium, phosphorus, sulfur, sodium, chlorine, magnesium, iodine and iron.**

2. Protein: contains 4 calories per gram. Provides the body nitrogen needs. Meat contains complete proteins while vegetables, fruits and nuts contain incomplete proteins. Protein is for the bones and muscles. It accounts to 50% of the bodies' needs. Must be eaten at every meal.

3.Carbohydrates: Contain 4 calories per gram. Body's preferable source of fuel. Good for energy. Three types of carbohydrates are monosachardies that are foods such as fruit, disaccharides are food such as milk or cane sugar, and polysaccharides are foods such as starches.

4.Fats: Building blocks for cell membranes, contributes to brain function, and hormones. The types of fats are saturated, unsaturated fats (monounsaturated and polyunsaturated) and trans-fat. Saturated fat and monounsaturated fats are easier to digest than polyunsaturated fats due to saturated and monounsaturated fats having short and medium chains and polyunsaturated fats having longer chains. High amounts of polyunsaturated fat is damaging and should be avoided. The types of polyunsaturated that are unnatural are in forms of canola oils and vegetable oils such as safflower and soy, and margarine. Medium and short chain foods are things like butter or coconut oil. Trans-fat the ingredient that makes the store life of a product last for years and should be avoided. Polyunsaturated fats are still essential to the body and should only be obtained from eating whole foods such as fish and nuts.

MEAL FREQUENCY AND TIMING MYTHS AND TRUTHS

Everyone now days is a little confused on how many meals one should eat during the day. People often have thoughts that if they eat a certain number of meals in a certain way at certain times that it's the way to go and doing it any other way will not confer them to have any results. Let me tell you right now the most important thing for fat loss and in the opposite case, weight gain, entirely depends how much food you eat in a day (of course what you eat too) and how active you are.

You can eat 10 meals in the day consisting of nothing but carrots and you will lose your weight (and by weight I mean muscle as well as fat and you'll look like an anorexic vogue model).

You can eat 2 meals in the day and eat the equivalent of a guy who just did two hot dog eating competitions and ate enough to feed the hulk and optimus prime combined and you WILL gain weight (and by weight I mean fat).

It doesn't even matter when you eat the meals with those following examples either. You intake more than you burn in a day you'll gain weight and vice versa. Also, as a no-brainer, if you eat complete junk for those meals it will wreck havoc to your hormones and organs and just like the study I said previously on the rats having good healthy fats vs the fats to avoid will determine how fast and how efficiently you'll either gain or lose the weight.

The argument is that if you eat every 3 hours and you eat 6 meals a day you would stoke the metabolic fire and thus lose weight plus you need protein every 3 hours otherwise your muscles would waste away. This is simply not the case.

There was a study done on healthy males where one group ate three meals, while the other ate 14. At the end of the study the group that ate the three meals had increased satiety (felt fuller) but they decreased their hunger cravings throughout the day. Plus their Resting **metabolic rate was increased** in the three meal group vs the 14 meal group. To top it off, it can help with glucose control for diabetics. Quoting the study: "Glucose and insulin profiles showed greater fluctuations, but a lower AUC of glucose in the LFr (low frequency) diet compared with the HFr (high frequency) diet". This means that the glucose ratings in the 3 meal group compared with the 14 meal group was actually lower. (17).

I would generally recommend one should have 3 meals. The reason is that you'll be able to have a much better chance of getting a variety of foods, hence you would get more nutrients to nourish your body efficently and vitamins. The least I would recommend for someone is to have two meals. The most I would recommend for someone trying to lose weight is again, 3 meals. If you wanted to gain weight then eating 6 meals will help. There's no science behind that, at least that I can see, but the benefits of eating that many meals to gain weight (and any meal number higher than 3) is that you have more opportunities to eat and you "train" your body to want more food by eating at specific times.

Meal timing

As mentioned meal timing is such a small thing compared to the amount taken during the day. We all have different lifestyles and ways to eat. So if you were to eat 3 meals and ate them at 11AM, 3PM, and 7:30PM or 1PM, 4PM, 9PM would it really matter? Not really. However if your goal was preformance and strength then yes it would matter to an extent to when you train. Personally I would advise someone to have a meal before they train. Preferably set the training at least 2 hours apart if it's a big meal and an hour if all your eating is a small snack (like fruits and some fish for instance). I also would advise to eat right after training since your body does need to replace what it has used for the exertion you put it through. So that means it is beneficial at this point to have carbohydrates to replenish energy (for the physiology inclined people, ATP stores), and replenish the damaged muscles with protein. Best type of carbohydrates to have at this point would be the monosaccharide type which is the fruits. So if you were to say have your first meal at 11AM go train at 3PM then right after training (we'll say 4PM is when you get home), have your next meal and make sure you have more fruits with this meal. Fruits I would recommend would be pineapple and papayas. They have digestive enzymes that help absorb protein (for instance, pineapple has bromelain), and these will surely speed up recovery.

So this is practically all you need to know about meal frequency and timing. Get all the nutrients and vitamins from a variety of only the best natural foods and eat when you are best able to eat. Stress while eating is actually a bigger thing to be concerned about when eating for the sole fact that if you are stressed you won't be able to digest your food properly as you should. So for all of you that are in such a rush to eat at a certain time you should just calm down first then eat. Eat when you have the time to finish and eat when you are in a happy environment when possible. Too often have I seen someone not "able to eat because they have no appetite" from being in a stressful environment such as a horned two headed monkey knawing on their arm and the other head yelling that one of their eyes is weird compared to the other whilst trying to eat a meal that they just forced themselves to eat at 6PM because they demanded themselves to eat at 6PM.

One final note on this is that I can understand that even if I presented the evidence that in fact eating less meals instead of 100 in a day will help with cravings I know that simply isn't the case if you just decided to ditch eating every 3 hours or however many meals you eat and decide to eat 3 meals a day instead. You have to understand your body has adapted to the routine of eating so very often and at specific times because you trained it to do so, that it's natural if you changed your meal patterns your body will respond by sending a craving to eat. The craving isn't exactly a strong craving to the point where you have to resort to eating your co-worker because he looks like a chicken (and for guys, a nice juicy steak with a skirt), but you'll feel it a little. You'll get over it very quickly in a week or two. My experience with myself and clients has been the case usually in this general time peroid. You actually look forward to having the next meal rather than it being a chore also. It's very simple to plan your lifestyle around this way too. If you are adamant that you like eating your 6-10 meals a day or eating every 3 hours then I'm not stopping you, but please know that they don't confer to any metabolic benefits by eating more, and eating more just basically means more opportunities in the day to eat.

30-DAY PALEO HABIT THREE

SIMPLIFY YOUR EATING, SIMPLIFY YOUR HEALTH

I want you to try, no matter how many meals you are eating right now just to get down to eating only three.

REASON FOR HABIT: By only eating three meals instead of more than three you will be forced to make a decision to actually eat healthy rather than just eat junk. Eating more will lead to more opportunities to eat and if you are eating more you have trained your body to expect food at certain times and your body is expecting to eat much more than it should. By eating less meals you teach your body to not require so many and thus control your hunger cravings. When you eat healthy for these three meals you also teach your body to only want the best and to not over-eat or binge on anything else. You will naturally eat less which means you will naturally lose weight.

Your MATH will serve as your RIFLE: The role of calories

Remember the baseline numbers we've been talking about at the first day of the 30 days? We will be using your lean body mass, if you have it, or your starting weight. I like to have lean body mass taken into account because it is a much more accurate way to see what your starting point is. This here is your rifle. Why? Because you now have a weapon which you can use! The weapon is YOUR numbers. To load the rifle all you need to do is do some calculations and find the final figure. To fire the rifle you just need to implement what you have found!

First we have to know how many calories are in a gram of protein, a carbohydrate, and a fat. **For protein and carbohydrates the calorie count is 4 and for fat the calorie count is 9.**

The second thing we have to do is find our "baseline" on calories. We need to know how much calories roughly we need to intake in order to maintain our weight and then decrease that value to start by 300-500 calories. There are many diets out there that claim results by limiting this or that macro nutrient, or by having a certain number of meals, but they all have one thing in common; they all try and force the person to eat less, hence less calories and hence weight loss.

To calculate your lean body mass if you have done the skin fold test via trainer or yourself via accumeasure skin caliper, you first write down your total weight and then write your total body fat percentage, you then minus the fat percentage from your total weight. So if I were 100kg (220 pounds) and I was 10% body fat which is 10% of 100kg is 10kg (22 pounds), we minus that from the total weight so our lean body mass now would be 100kg minus 10kg equals 90kg (198 pounds).

Next you'd want to figure out your total daily energy expenditure (TDEE). To do this you'll need to find out your RMR which is your resting metabolic rate and your physical activity level (PAL).

Now before I lose you, let me explain what these are.

TDEE = means how much energy you expend in a day

RMR = means how much energy you expend during rest. That means things such as your body just simply rebuilding tissue for instance or your organs working. Yes you are indeed burning calories just sitting down also.

PAL = Physical activity! Exercise! The more active you are the more calories you burn

With all that said, let's get down to calculating your caloric needs.

Miffin formula for calculating RMR

The one problem with this calculation is it only intakes bodyweight. It's good if you may be a bit obese but it's definitely not as accurate as having your body fat checked. You will have to do some fine-tuning so please do keep that in mind. The formula is as follows:

MALES:

RMR = (10 x weight in kg) + (6.25 x height in cm) – (5 x age) + 5

FEMALES:

RMR = (10 x weight in kg) + (6.25 x height in cm) – (5 x age) + 161

Katch McArdle formula

This is more accurate since it takes into account lean body mass and not just overall body mass.

RMR = 370 + 21.6 x lean mass in kg

Once you have figured out your RMR it's time to calculate your TDEE. The formula for that is the following as provided by Harris J. Bemedict F. A study of basal metabolism in man:

Sedentary (little or no exercise): RMR x 1.2

Lightly active (light exercise 1-3 days a week) RMR x 1.375

Moderately active (moderate exercise/sports 3-5 days per week) RMR 1.55

Very active (Hard exercise/sports 6-7 days per week) RMR 1.725

Extra active (Very hard daily exercise/sports and physical job or training 2 x daily) RMR x 1.9

Lets take an example of that same 100kg man we had earlier into this equation. He has 90kg worth of mass. He uses the katch McArdle formula. 370 + 21.6 x 90 = 2314.

We find out that he is extra active. By this definition it is because he works in a labor intensive job daily, goes to the gym 3 times a week and does kick boxing 3 times a week for a good hour and trains hard and not just sitting and talking. Therefore we calculate his RMR x 1.9 which is 2314 x 1.9 = 4396.6 calories.

Now all he has to do is subtract 300-500 calories from his meal planning and achieve fat loss! It's that simple! If he isn't losing weight from simply subtracting the 500 calories (which I doubt with that level of activity anyway), all he has to do is decrease it by 100 extra for the entire week then check if he is. If the answer is no then further decrease it and repeat the cycle until he is.

As you can see from counting your calories you now have a good guide on how to lose fat and aren't in the dark about it either. This is a sure thing and when you have nothing to work with by just aimlessly trying a diet with a great name and starving yourself you in the dark!

How to plan your meals

The next step is planning your meals. The first thing you have to do is weigh your food by your digital weight scale (a normal food weighing scale will do too). Remember to note when you measure your food if it's cooked or uncooked.

The next thing is to go to an online database and find out how much calories each of your food has. At first it may seem a little daunting but when you have the knowledge for the food you don't have to keep checking each and every time.

Some of the best websites to check your food are:

HTTP://www.Calorieking.com.au

www.nal.usda.gov/finc/foodcomp/search

www.caloriecount.com

www.fitday.com/webfit/index.html

www.nutritiondata.com

When you have your meals you ideally want one protein source, one carbohydrate source and a vegetable source. You can have as much vegetables as you like. Protein should be had with every meal and do not cut the fat out of the meat since they contain nutrients as well as to help you feel fuller. Carbohydrates will come from your vegetables, fruits and nuts.

As mentioned in the benefits of paleo section a rule of thumb is it is best to eat your vegetables and meat first and your carbohydrates last because this way it'll help you not to overeat since the vegetables and meat are much more filling than the carbohydrates. Think of your carbohydrates like a desert if you will. Also it will help diabetics have better glycemic control (10).

Let's do a sample meal plan for someone who eats 3 meals a day, has a total daily requirement of 3000 calories to maintain weight and wants to lose weight so will cut the calories by 500, making it 2500.

The scenario is that he likes having big meals (and particularly breakfast), but likes his dinner to be smallest, so we'll evenly spread the total calories for each of his meals with that in mind. That will equate to 833.33 calories roughly per meal. We will use calorieking.com.au for the measurements.

Breakfast can be the following:

A 250gram lean sirloin steak, grilled (405 calories)

Three 50gram Whole hard boiled eggs (183 calories)

One cup of broccoli (48 calories)

One large apple (106 calories) and one large banana (122 calories)

TOTAL CALORIES FOR MEAL ONE = 864

Lunch time meal:

250grams Fresh salmon (baked)

15 raw almonds (108 calories)

2 cups fresh mashed papaya (156 calories)

TOTAL CALORIES FOR MEAL TWO = 854

Dinner meal

250gram lobster, boiled (243 calories)

Traditional fried eggs (2 large whole raw egg = 144 calories and 102 calories butter used 250.8 calories)

12 boiled asparagus spears (60 calories)

5 medium raw macadamia nuts (125 calories)

1 cup of raspberries (54 calories)

TOTAL CALORIES FOR MEAL 3 = 732.8

TOTAL CALORIES FOR MEALS OF THE DAY = 2450 CALORIES

Now we have a total map out of what to eat for one of the days of the week. Of course this is just an example. You can have different meal plans if you desire for other days or if you like the plan you have now you can simply stick with it or replace one thing with something else and calculate the calories (like replacing a banana with another apple or orange etc.) You can use any other foods, and recipes you desire, have two big meals and one snack, have a bigger dinner etc. Plan it to how you like it and how you see fit for your lifestyle.

30 DAY PALEO HABIT FOUR
<u>**YOU SET THE COURSE! NOW SAIL IT!**</u> For 30 days you will stick to the meal plans in which you set out for yourself. **REASON FOR HABIT: Just writing something on paper is one thing, but actually doing it is another. You mapped out how to get to your destination so now all you have to do is follow it and get to where you want to be!**

Your hands and thumb will serve as your body armor: the role of portion control

So now that we've got the calories down to the pat in terms of meal plans what happens when you are forced to not be able to measure a serving of protein, carbohydrates, or fats without your usual tools? Not to worry that's where your hand is your trust worthy body armor!

Everyone's hand, yes I am aware, doesn't change in size, but that's perfect FOR YOU. To measure a serving of protein all you have to simply do is close your fist. To measure a serving of carbohydrates all you have to simply do is use the palm of your hand. Finally, to measure a serving of fat all you have to simply do is measure it by the outline of your thumb (where the tip of your thumb to the first line, which is the center of your thumb). These translate into a cup for protein and carbohydrates and a teaspoon for your fats.

Let's put this into practice. Let's say you're invited to an Asian restaurant for dinner. Your usual dinner consists of 500 calories in total. You know that protein and carbohydrates equal 4 calories and fats equal 9. You decide to get a plate of shrimp, and since you decide to treat yourself a little bit since it's after a workout and there are vegetables there, you decide to get a stir fry consisting of mixed vegetables and rice. So shrimp and rice mixed with vegetables for your first plate. A serve of protein is usually 30 grams and a serve of carbohydrates is usually 40 grams (one cup to each). If we do the math, the estimate if you used your palm of your hand and fist as an estimate would be that you would have 120 calories for the protein and 160 calories for the carbohydrates, and maybe a little extra for the vegetables (say 15 calories). If we don't take the vegetables mixed in the rice the total calorie count for your plate would be 280 calories! You now know how much you need to eat for your 2nd plate! Of course this is purely an educated estimate but an educated estimate is much better than just turning off the light, holding a knife, and taking a stab in the dark! Chances are, if you know already how much calories this and that has from your own meal plans, you'd be more than likely to be bang on target.

As you can see portion control is a safe guard in any special occasion or if you were to go on a road trip. It serves as your body armor so you can have a body that just plain looks like body armor by not over-eating and sticking to your plan!

CLIFF NOTES FOR THE CONFUSED AND IMPATIENT

CHAPTER THREE PART TWO

1. Meal frequency and habit three: Eating more meals does not offer metabolic benefits and eating every 3 hours is not necessary. Eating less frequently actually does offer benefits in terms of glucose control and feeling full and in fact, resting metabolic can go up with only 3 meals a day. The habit for these 30 days is to eat only 3 meals a day.

2.Find out how much to eat via calories: We need to find out your TDEE (total daily energy expenditure), RMR (resting metabolic rate), and PAL (physical activity level) which will indicate how many calories you need to maintain your weight. Then from that we will subtract 500 calories from your daily meals and hence the weight loss will commence! The miffin formula takes into account only weight if you didn't measure your LBM by measuring body fat by a fitness professional or an accumeasure skin fold caliper.

3.Miffin formula for calculating RMR: MALES: RMR = (10 x weight in kg) + (6.25 x height in cm) – (5 x age) + 5

FEMALES: RMR = (10 x weight in kg) + (6.25 x height in cm) – (5 x age) + 161

4.Katch McArdle formula: RMR = 370 + 21.6 x lean mass in kg (this is if you have LBM, lean body mass, figure)

5.Calculate TDEE: Sedentary (little or no exercise): RMR x 1.2

Lightly active (light exercise 1-3 days a week) RMR x 1.375

Moderately active (moderate exercise/sports 3-5 days per week) RMR 1.55

Very active (Hard exercise/sports 6-7 days per week) RMR 1.725

Extra active (Very hard daily exercise/sports and physical job or training 2 x daily) RMR x 1.9

6.How to plan your meals: Subtract 500 calories from the figure you have obtained. Now make each meal even with the number of calories (E.G. 3000 is your maintenance figure so, minus 500 is 2500. 2500 divided by three equals 833.33). Make sure you have protein at every meal and have a vegetable source. Find out the calories your meal will have by calculating the serving sizes of foods by calorie websites such as: Calorieking.com.au or caloriecount.com

7.Portion control: A fist is the serving size of protein, a palm of the hand is the serving size of carbohydrates and your thumb is a serving size of fat.

8.Habit four: Follow the meal plan you have set for yourself.

BRAVING THE SUPERMARKET SHELVES AND AVOIDING THE INGREDIENT LAND MINES

This will be the last thing you'll need to know in terms of how to select food. You've already got the knowledge in how much to eat and how to use the food to lose the fat. This can practically be a book in itself but fear not you will get a basic run down on the ingredients to avoid in the foods you decide to buy. Avoid these land mines and you'll be safe on the other side of your health.

Ingredients to avoid in food

Soy

Surprised this is on the list? Soy over the years has been thought to be healthy for us. We have been told it can let us have great cardiovascular effects and it can help with your lipid profile (which means cholesterol and triglycerides, and in turn reduce your risk for heart diseases), also that it can help with bones.

There are many other benefits been told I'm sure but these three, however, are the main benefits I have always heard. Soy doesn't show any increase in lipid profile or cardiovascular benefits (18), nor does soy isoflavones have any bone sparring effect (19).

Soy is mostly used as filler and soy raises estrogen levels (20). High estrogen levels for females and men can raise an abundance of problems and health issues. As an example men can expect to experience libido issues and that means erectile dysfunction (21)! I certainly for one like to have a working Lo Wang, todger… whatever you want to call it.

You would be surprised how many food products have soy. Even a can of tuna can have soy!

Soy can go by other names such as: Guar gum, Lecithin, protein extender, HVP (Hydrolyzed vegetable protein), Vegetable broth or starch, textured vegetable protein (TVP) and even disguised in the ingredients as protein. Beware of bulking agent and emulsifier also.

MSG also known as monosodium glutamate

Monosodium glutamate (MSG) is used as a flavor-enhancer and is most commonly found in processed foods. This is a very common ingredient I'm sure everyone has heard and seen. MSG is a toxic substance that kills the nerve cells of the body. This is a bad thing because we need our nerves to function. From our brain, moving our hands and to our heart continuing to beat. MSG is also known to make one's appetite for food larger than normal which means that one can overeat much more easier. Neurological disorders along with overeating are more than good enough reasons to dismiss this.

"At 3, 30, or 300 µM MSG, the percentage of cell death was approximately 25%, ~40%, or 50%". After years of damaging your nerves with MSG you would do well to take vitamin C as Vitamin C has been shown to help reduce the MSG damage of neurons (22).

Artificial sweeteners; Aspartame, Saccharin, and Sucralose

The big 3 in the artificial sweetener world are these. Remember a simple word and you'll know to avoid them. ASS. Don't make an ASS of yourself and you'll be well on your way to good health!

These artificial sweeteners have some of the same effects of MSG. In fact, artificial sweeteners such as Aspartame have been shown as a possible link to some cancers (23). To top that off, you know that diet sodas or energy drinks you're so fond of? Aspartame in high dosages can cause seizures and that goes for people that haven't previously had a seizure either (24). Artificial sweeteners are just what they sound like; they are artificial sweeteners to make the food taste sweet. That muffin you had that had zero sugar but tasted very sweet? Most likely it had one of these. There is much more associated risks with these types of sweeteners so I would definitely avoid these at all cost.

As a side note, splenda, in the health and fitness world has been deemed a healthy substitute to the bad effects of these products. Sucralose is found as splenda and once again mostly processed foods contain it.

Sugar

Sugar is addictive. White sugar can cause a number of health issues and it is believed that it can even deprive the body of nutrients! Sugar is so addictive in fact that in one study that I have read 2 rats had either cocaine or sugar. The rat that had the sugar was the rat that got addicted to it the fastest! (25) Maybe for humans that's a bit extreme to say that those refined sugar ingredients you see in our foods it's on the same level of cocaine but I will state it's not so unbelievable that it can almost be borderline drug abuse to a lot of individuals. Take kids for an example. Haven't you ever seen the biggest tantrum in the stores or a fast food place when a kid doesn't get the cake or chocolate Sunday? Or how about adults getting wild mood swings and hostile when you tell them to stop eating such sweets and food laden with sugar when they have eaten the stuff for years?

Sugar plagues a lot of our foods. The chocolate in the isles and all the sweets and foods for kids are the best example. It's one, if not the first ingredient of many on the list! People do have sugar withdrawals because they have been craving for it after years and years of being addicted to sweet foods. It's obvious to see how this can lead to diabetes and obesity with the over consumption when you eat yourself to an early grave by this ingredient's taste.

Sodium Nitrate and Sodium Nitrite

Notice the letter I and the letter A in both words after sodium. No I didn't spell the same word! These are the chemicals used to preserve meat. Just like how trans-fat may preserve butter or margarine, this is their brother. A lot of studies done on meat in particular have said that the meat causes one to have an increased risk of cancer. It's easy to dismiss it on being purely just because of poor cooking habits and saturated fat or whatever else they claim it to be but one of the main reasons are these. It is shown that these ingredients actually may be carcinogenic and in turn can lead to cancer (26). Stick to grass-fed unprocessed meats.

Recombinant bovine growth hormone

Sticking with the things that go into our meat, this ingredient (rBGH), is what makes our cattle grow fast. It is a growth hormone that farmers use to increase their production of cows such as milk production. rBGH milk contains high quantities of insulin growth like factor (IGF-1) which is a hormone that we all have. But unnatural levels of this hormone can be shown to have cancers that are namely associated with the risk of eating meat in the media such as prostate and colon cancers. It can even be linked to breast cancers (27).

Trans-fat

As a recap on the section that we had on fats, this is the fat to avoid. It is the ingredient that has anything spelt with "hydro" in it. It is used to increase shelf life of products such as margarine and butter. It can lead to clogged arteries and heart diseases. A example of the trans-fat in food with the word hydro in it is an ingredient called hydrogenated vegetable oil. Be aware that it isn't necessary to actually put trans-fat in the nutrition label section of the food you eat, but it is necessary to say that it has trans-fat as an ingredient in it. This is how you find it.

Refined vegetable oil

You must be careful of the oils you see on the shelf. Namely soybean oil, corn oil, safflower oil, canola oil and peanut oil. These are all classed as refined vegetable oils. Don't let the word vegetable fool you! Remember what we discussed before about long chained fats? Having an excess of long chained fats is what causes inflammation to the body. These oils will cause the excess.

These are made with chemical and mechanical processes used to extract the oil from seeds. They use high temperatures and chemical solvents and deodorize and bleach them. All the minerals that you know are good for you in the vegetables and nuts are gone and all that is left is a bottle full of liquid that can cause free-radicals running through your body. It can also mean it can cause damage to your DNA and impair your insulin response which means that you'll have problems with losing weight and getting the most out of your foods. Omega-6, while our body does need it, vegetable oils causes an excessive amount of it which can negate the effects of omega-3s in your daily eating habits and is also linked to a number of health problems that once again we hear associated with fat intake. The process to create refined vegetable oils is the same that creates trans-fat. Vegetable oils are known to contribute to cancers and heart disease.

Potassium Bromate

This is used to increase the volume of breads rolls and flours. Just like the cows being pumped full of growth hormone this can be shown to increase the likely hood of cancer in persons consuming. Our endocrine system is a very important system that regulates our hormones. This ingredient is shown to cause negative effects on the endocrine system (28, 29). When your hormones are not optimal you can expect almost every kind of issue known. A good tip is that melatonin might help a little with suppressing some of this ingredient's negative effects (29).

AKA And Artificial coloring

AKA is the stuff that is used in beverages, candy, cereal, energy bars, puddings, deli meat, frostings, fast food, ice cream, and even meat and fish! Ever wonder why the meat and fish look fresh? This is the ingredient to make it look so.

It also comes in these names: FD&C Blue #1, Bright blue, Blue #2, Caramel color, Erythrosine, Yellow 5 & 6, Fast green, Sea green, Allura Red, Royal blue, Ingtotine and more. If you see any color for an ingredient you know this is it.

As a little detour story of this in action I when I was in Philippines I went to a fish market and I luckily had a friend that warned me to be careful not to purchase fish from that particular market and be wary of others. I asked him exactly why. He said to me to look at the eyes, and ask myself why the eyes were so fresh-looking despite the fish being there for more than a few days. Seeing as I didn't want to have any worms or ruin my vacation of having the worst toilet time in history doing the sign of the cross and promising the big man upstairs to build 5 churches in his honor if this pain would just go…I took heed and went to buy fish that had the blood red eyes but were just freshly caught. So a good tip is not just to look at the fish and see if it is unnaturally fresh looking but the eyes also, should you be at a supermarket in the east or west.

High fructose corn syrup (HFCS)

Corn starch that is separated from the kernel and converted into corn syrup is the definition of this ingredient. It is used as a sweetener. It's made from genetically-modified corn and can be shown to cause problems such as cardiovascular diseases, obesity, arthritis, insulin resistance, and raised LDL cholesterol (30).

This can also be known as the following: Corn, corn sugar, corn syrup, cornstarch, crystalline fructose/glucose, dextrose, corn syrup solids, glucose, glucose syrup, lecithin from corn and maltodextrin.

Refined Wheat

Refined wheat can be shown to cause discomfort to the gastrointestinal tract and digestive system as a whole. Wheat contains traces of gluten just like grains and that can mean you can experience tiredness, bloating, and in some cases diarrhea (31).

What you want to be aware of are these: Gluten, gelatinized starch, starch, triticale, vegetable gum/starch, vital fluten, wheat bran, wheat germ, wheat gluten, wheat malt, wheat starch, gum Arabic, triticum aestivum.

Keep in mind that most grains actually have traces of gluten and is more reason why we don't include them in this plaeo plan.

Pasteurized, homogenized and UHT milk

While I am aware that this isn't really an ingredient, and it's just food I feel compelled to include this here in this section for last. Not many people know the differences of each of these.

Pasteurized milk is a method originally made to help prevent people from having health problems from drinking raw milk from cows. When a cow is mistreated, not raised properly and you drink it's milk raw then you WILL catch life-threatening bacteria and especially if you drink the milk from a diseased cow. In this process, one heats up the milk to kill of the bacteria in the milk. The problem is that doing this will get rid of most of the good things in the milk too and enzymes such as lactase needed to digest milk in those lactose intolerant. You aren't really getting anything out of the milk except some vitamins so it's best to save your money on other food that you can benefit more from.

Homogenized milk is chemically altering the fat globule of the milk to make it creamy. Anything that is chemically modified is obviously out. There might or might not be any studies to indicate what problems this can cause but I say to stay away just from the fact it's chemically altered.

UHT stands for ultra high treated milk. This is a process where, just as it sounds, they treat the milk at ultra high temperatures and do a number of other things to ensure the shelf life of the milk is extended. Once something is extended beyond it's capacity, you don't want that running through your system.

In fact you'll notice that in diary there is traces of pasteurized milk as one of it's ingredients.

If you absolutely must have diary and you want to deter a little from this plan I would say if you stick to something grass-fed, be sure to be aware of the source in which your food comes from (make sure the cattle is clean, healthy and raised well) and make sure that they aren't injected with hormones as well as making sure the food is as unprocessed as possible (raw) then 3 servings per day MAX doesn't really lead to any health complications per se. It is when it is used eaten in excess and when what you eat is unnatural that it can do things like increase hormones (IGF-1) to unnatural levels and cause cancer.

One last note; if you buy the yogurt in the shelves thinking you'll improve your gut health by it's pro-biotic properties then consider that most of the yogurt in the store is more than likely to be processed already and by it's transport to get there the good bacteria might already be dead. Best bet is to look into investing in something called kefir and making your own pro-biotic by growing them from raw milk if possible.

There might be an abundance more of ingredients that I haven't mentioned and no doubt there will always be new ones coming out in the near future. The best thought process I can offer you to defend yourselves against these ingredients is this: **if you don't know how an ingredient is made or even what it is, no matter if anyone claims it to be healthy with a tick with a heart symbol you shouldn't ingest it.**

30 DAY PALEO HABIT FIVE

<u>WATCH YOUR STEP! DON'T FALL ON THE TRIPWIRE!</u>

For 30 days you will aim to avoid the ingredients in this book and ingredients that you do not know.

REASON FOR HABIT: In the start when losing fat you might be inclined to put sauces and other various condiments or go for the tastier alternative to food that you consider healthy. Losing the fat by controlling what you eat is hard enough to begin with but now that you have that down, it's time to take the next step and improve your health as well as help your fat loss more by mastering your taste buds just that bit more by avoiding these harmful ingredients in your food.

Nutritional considerations for diabetics

Following this plan where you cut out the starches and only eat fruit and vegetables is a huge step in ensuring you have better glycemic control. Eating the vegetables and meat first before you eat the fruit or a carbohydrate treat as well as using portion control, especially on carbohydrates, further ensures this.

If you were to eat heaps of fruit or you were to have carbohydrate treats here and there, my best suggestion is to time those treats and fruits around the time you train. Our body is more able to handle carbohydrates well after a hard training session because we have depleted our carbohydrate stores and our body is asking us to replenish.

Also keep in mind that you still want to have some candy and jelly beans on hand when you train. Why? It's insurance. Yes I am aware it's not paleo and I am aware that it might be loaded with bad ingredients but these sweets can save your life. If you get down to dangerously low sugar levels, as a diabetic it can be potentially fatal. So please, even though you take pride in this plan, it is allowed to have something to save your life.

If you are having really bad results with controlling your sugar levels with 3 meals then experiment with the number that is right for you. Personally, I haven't heard any diabetic having a major problem with 3 meals but if you are one of them then try 4 and so on.

Nutritional considerations for pro-athletes

Pro-athletes train as if it was their full time job and how can they expected to have all their calories just from meat, fruit and veggies alone? Simple! They can't! If you are an athlete, especially one that trains 5-8 hours a day, I would suggest now adding starches to your meals instead of takeaways with bad ingredients. Yes I am aware there is gluten in some grains but you are getting nutrition from them (e.g. Phosphorus from the oats, and oats actually doesn't have gluten content like wheat does). Remember that starches contain many chains of sugars, and it is perfect for fattening up someone. Super high energy food is a must for athletes along with nutrition. In this case, I would recommend still having meat, having the fruit too, and some vegetables (have this last because vegetables can deter your appetite and you need to eat!) and having carbohydrates from other sources. Carbohydrates are the bodies' preferred fuel source and athletes need the energy more than anyone. If you aren't someone that trains more than 4 hours a day like it was your job then stick to not including them. Also remember to drink plenty of water. Last thing for athletes is it is advisable to eat more meals purely because you cannot get all your nutritional requirements in 3, unless, like me, you can eat a planet in a sitting all 3 of your meals.

Nutritional considerations for pregnant women

Now before you ladies shoot me down and tell me I'm a man and I know nothing of the troubles of pregnancy, and you're right, I don't in terms of how it feels, I still can offer some advice!

I realize that you are all more hungry and that you might have cravings for certain foods and abolish others. Well I say fine. Plan your calorie count and meals around those. How many extra calories do you need to support that miracle inside you? I would say you would need no more than 500 tops over your maintenance, 250 being the sweet point, and please don't think about losing weight when having a baby. You want this baby to be strong right? So focus on just maintaining the body-fat to a reasonable level and think about losing that fat (whatever you gained) AFTER.

In terms of keeping the baby healthy, you would be wise to avoid the ingredients I listed, avoid alcohol, avoid smoking and drugs. I realize that enough is common sense but I can't stress it enough.

If you are one of those types that just wants something sweet I'd suggest to have RAW honey (not the one you get in the super market shelves that is absolutely loaded with ingredients like high fructose corn syrup!). I realize it isn't "paleo" but I want you to beat the cravings in the healthiest way you can manage and not pile on the weight by binging on bad things. Honey is very sweet and you can use it on whatever it is you want to make sweet. If you wanted chocolate you can buy chocolate butters and use that on something to make it tasty.

Don't eat anything you'd be allergic to and also avoid spicy food and if you can caffeine. These increase your metabolic rate and right now you need and your body is already stressed enough by taking care of the child and you. Drink plenty of water also.

Although this is a nutrition section I'll say something a little about exercise. In terms of exercise, don't do any exercises that are "jerky" or "explosive" such as jumping or running. Instead go for a bike ride or even swim. Be careful of your center of gravity too since you have that child in front of you so don't do any exercises like clean and presses at the gym. Don't do exercises lying on your back either, make sure you are either seated or standing, This ensures the baby's safety. Some recommendations are shadow boxing, swimming, biking, you can do weights but be aware what could be potentially dangerous, elliptical trainer and some bodyweight movements (like nice controlled squats but NOT push ups). I would say go easier than you are used to with training instead of training to hard. Keeping active is fine but if you were to be pregnant don't expect to train for the Olympics while pregnant! Low impact exercises over high impact exercises is a good rule to follow.

Remember, it's about keeping your body-fat reasonable to what it normally was before your pregnancy so you won't have much fat to lose later on. You won't get a ripped 8-pack while pregnant, not only is that dangerous for you and the baby, but it's unrealistic.

CLIFF NOTES FOR THE CONFUSED AND IMPATIENT

CHAPTER THREE PART THREE

1. Ingredients to avoid:

Soy: Increases estrogen and does not provide cardiovascular benefits or bone sparring.

Goes by other names such as Guar gum, Lecithin, protein extender, HVP (Hydrolyzed vegetable protein), Vegetable broth or starch, textured vegetable protein

(TVP) and even disguised in the ingredients as protein. Beware of bulking agent and emulsifier also.

MSG: Kills nerves, makes appetite bigger. Vitamin C is shown to help reduce damage to neurons from MSG.

Aspartame, Saccharin, Sucralose (artificial sweeteners): can cause seizures, and can be a possible link to cancer. This is used to make drinks and other foods taste sweet. Remember the acronym A.S.S to remember these three.

Sugar: Not only is it addictive to ingest (makes everything sweet), and is one of the causes of health issues such as diabetes and obesity.

Sodium nitrate and sodium nitrite: These are the ingredients that preserve meat. It is linked to cancers.

Recombinant bovine growth hormone (rBGH): Used to increase cattle size and dairy production in cattle such as milk which can lead to unnaturally increased IGF-1 and in turn can lead to ailments such as breast cancers.

Trans-fat: you find this ingredient by any word containing "hydro" in it such as hydrogenated vegetable oil. This is what trans-fat is. It is what makes the products on the shelves last 10 years or how ever long. These can clog your arteries.

Refined vegetable oil: These are unnaturally high in polyunsaturated fats and can cause free-radical damage in your body.

Potassium Bromate: Used to increase volume in pastries. Shown to disrupt the endocrine system (which means it'll wreck havoc on your hormones). Melatonin helps with suppressing it's negative effects.

AKA and artificial coloring: Used to make the meat look fresh when it is days old.

High fructose corn syrup (HFCS): used as a sweetener and can be linked to insulin resistance, diabetes, obesity, arthritis, rises in LDL cholesterol and cardiovascular diseases. This can also be known as the following: Corn, corn sugar, corn syrup, cornstarch, crystalline fructose/glucose, dextrose, corn syrup solids, glucose, glucose syrup, lecithin from corn and maltodextrin.

Refined wheat: Wrecks havoc in your gastrointestinal track. What you want to be aware of are these: Gluten, gelatinized starch, starch, triticale, vegetable gum/starch, vital fluten, wheat bran, wheat germ, wheat gluten, wheat malt, wheat starch, gum Arabic, triticum aestivum.

Pasteurized, homogenized and UHT milk: Pasteurized is boiling it to high temperatures, homogenized is chemically altering the fat globules and UHT stands for ultra high treated milk which is to increase shelf life.

2. Habit five: Avoid the ingredients listed in food.

3. Nutritional considerations for diabetics: have candy or a jelly bean in handy with you when you train for insurance. Eat vegetables and protein first before you eat carbohydrates.

4. Nutritional considerations for athletes: It is OK to have starches when your full time job is training all day. Eat more meals.

5. Nutritional considerations for pregnant women: Your calories should be extra to what you are eating to nourish the baby but do not exceed 500 calories. Don't focus on weight loss but focus on keeping your weight reasonable. If you crave some foods that you can't just shake no matter what, then plan those foods by keeping a tally of calories. If you have a sweet tooth, add honey to your meals. Avoid caffeine, alcohol and spicy foods. Lay off the drugs and tobacco. Don't do exercises that cause you to lay on your back or to harm the baby, keep in mind the gravity of your weight that is in front of you so be careful not to do any explosive movements too. Things like crunches and push ups from the floor are out. Low impact over high impact exercises.

Armed with success!

Now that you have all that's needed with nutrition you can ensure that you are on the right track when it comes to how much to eat in order to lose fat. Having a target and having a blueprint is what leads to success. This is half the battle done and this is the hardest. The next step is having the tools on how to train to have the other 50% ensured for your success!

CHAPTER 4: All things training all things results

"Be true to the game, because the game will be true to you. If you try to shortcut the game, then the game will shortcut you. If you put forth the effort, good things will be bestowed upon you. That's truly about the game, and in some ways that's true about life too." - Micheal Jordan

Before we get into the how-to with training we have to get into the mindset of what it takes to get these results. Don't dismiss this as something that's not useful because this is the most useful tool that you must have. I'm sure you've seen time after time the same people who look the same year after year don't you? The mindset is the ultimate factor as to why they do look the way they do year after year. It's one thing just to get up off your bed and go for a run, lift weights, or whatever exercise you choose, and say you did something, yet it's an entirely different thing to get up off your bed do the chosen activity you want to do as exercise but instead of just doing it, you know that it's a fight, a struggle and a war. It's you against you! Let me explain.

You have to keep improving no matter what it is you choose to do! This is the secret! You have to work as hard as you possibly can and give it all you have without being comfortable until the session is over. Don't be one of those people that jog for 30 minutes just for the sake of doing it, but be one of those people that try jog as fast as you possibly can and try cover much more distance in 30 minutes than you did the last time you decided to jog.

Every time you train, it is one step closer to your goals, and every time you improve you are making your body more desirable to what you want it to be. Every time you train it's not a chore, it's a reflection on how much you want it and in turn, your body will be a reflection and testament to your hard work and will.

Yes the training will be intense, yes it will take hard work, and yes there is no ways around it if you really want that body you desire, but just like your eating, this is something that you can control. You can do ANY exercise or ANY type of training, but if you do not put in the hard work as well as consistency for the long haul, you will never get the results you seek. So let's see what you can do and just how much you want your dream body! Let's not just get up out of where we are sitting, but let's stand and walk tall and get ready for this opportunity to let our body be a testament to our own will! Let's get in there and let's (expletive) do it!

The training philosophy

I know that this book is more about nutrition and it'll require a much bigger book to be more detailed on exercises to do. After all you brought this book in knowledge it was a diet plan, but what plan would be complete without a component on how to train? This philosophy will take you very far with all your training endeavors but just know before you implement it to please seek medical advice to know if you are healthy and good to do the exercise component of this program. You already did for your nutrition did you? I'd hate to see you hurt yourself so please do take care. So you are robust and healthy you say? Then here are the principles that I know will work and why!

1.Do as much as you can do in a time frame you set

What this means is, you have to set a deadline in regards to time of the training session and you do the exercises you choose as much as you can, as fast as you can, as properly as you can, for that time. No resting, no slouching! An example can be doing squats (whether bodyweight only or weighted, it's your choice) for 10 repetitions and doing push ups or barbell overhead presses for 10 repetitions for 10 minutes. Another example can be doing 50 yard sprints and 5 burpees for 10 minutes. You go at your own pace with these but you make sure you put in the effort to actually do as much as you can! There's no possible way you won't sweat, you will work every part of your body, and from the amount of work, burn off all the fat if you keep improving and working at it!

2.Keep a log book of your sessions

If you don't keep track of things and have a blueprint, then how will you know where to go? What writing down your sessions does is see where you are improving, where you are weakest, and how far you've come. Not only is this a tool for motivation (since it sure is motivating to see how much more fitter and stronger you are months after you re-visit an old workout you did), but this serves as a your rival. You WANT TO BEAT THIS CREATURE! YOU MUST BEAT THIS CREATURE! You look in your book to what you did Monday...You see that it took you 20 minutes to do 100 push ups and 100 squats. This fudge on a stick is taunting you. It's belittling you and it's belittling your ancestors! What's that I hear? Oh hell-est to the no-est! It just slipped a "your mom" and "your dad" joke! It's saying you can't possibly get 100 push ups and 100 squats in less time than what you did before, which was 20 minutes! Are you seriously going to take that? Well are ya? Huh? No? I thought so! Get in there, and show that potate (which is potato, but I don't want any paleo guys hounding me that I called their workout journals something starchy), that you'll beat this crustation to it's crust and get it done in even one second faster than you did before! Too right you will!

3.Do exercises that uses the whole body

To get the most work done in the shortest amount of time and get the best results you already know you have to work hard. It is the exercises that most people hate that are always the most results producing. They all have one thing in common. The exercises involve every single part of your body to work in order to complete the exercise. Doing bicep curls in a machine where you can sit down versus doing squats with a barbell on your back. Which of these two uses more muscles and which is more harder to accomplish one repetition? The squat of course! If you were a bodyweight enthusiast how about jogging lightly for thirty minutes versus doing burpees for thirty minutes? Of course the burpees. If you combine doing exercises that demand a whole body effort with doing it as fast as you can in a certain time frame you can see now how the fat will just melt off. For instance, if you lightly jog and used the philosophy of doing as much work in as little time, it's not a light jog anymore is it? It's a sprint and you'll be working every part of your body that much more. If you were just casually doing push ups within your comfort zone and stopping well before your body just had to and used the philosophy mentioned above, you'll not just be working your chest and arms, but the very act of holding yourself up at the very top position, breathing, and struggling to get more and more is an awesome core workout and will work your legs too! Don't believe me? Try holding yourself up in the top of the push-up position for as long as you can until you just cannot do it anymore. As a good challenge try aim to hold yourself up there for 10 minutes whilst keeping your back straight and not sagging it.

Here is a list of some exercises for people that are without a gym or with a gym that I know are effective for fat loss in a short period of time:

Best bodyweight exercises

Burpees

Squats

Lunges

Push ups

Mountain jumpers AKA Squat thrusts

Mountain climbers

Bear crawls AKA commando crawls

Crab walks

Duck walks

Alligator walks

Star jumps

Jumps in every variation e.g. Forward jumps, jumping on top of something

Pull-ups and chin-ups

Dips

Planks

Ab wheel

Skipping

Sprinting

Best exercises with weights

Squats

Barbell Dead lift

Over head presses

Weighted bodyweight exercises e.g. Bear crawls with back pack, chin ups with weight around waist etc.

Dumbbell farmer carries

Dumbbell dead lifts

Kettle bell swings

Barbell and dumbbell rows

Dumbbell snatches

Russian twists

This is a list of the basics and the tried and true exercises that will produce the best results. As a few are aware I excluded lifts that are complicated such as Olympic lifts for the fact that you'll more than likely injure yourself unless you are taught by a professional and have the necessary mobility on how to do them, and practice them for YEARS, not months. So all you have to do as the reader, and the doer, is pick 1-3 exercises from the list, whether weighted or unweighted, and work hard at them for the day. Write down your workout and keep trying to improve on it by repetitions or putting more weight on the bar when ready.

4. Train everyday

If you want the best results in the shortest amount of time I'm a big believer in training everyday but at the same time you should be well aware of your body. If you are very fatigued and very sore then it makes sense you don't push as hard the next day but you should at least do something and give it your best for that day. So as an example if you had a killer session worthy of being passed down to generations and you were quite literally so fatigued and sore the next day that just sitting down is a mission then I would advise you would do something such as go for a nice swim or to walk at a nice fast pace. Maybe you had a day where you went for all you got and more and surprisingly the next day you felt phenomenal, then what do you do? Go for it again! When your body says it needs to take it easy, then take it easy. In turn you'll know that sleeping and eating the right foods to nourish your body for another awesome workout is how you continue to make progress.

5.Always do something different

A good way to let the body keep obtaining results and for you to continue to remain motivated is to keep doing something different and what you want to do every time you train. Remember, the key is giving it your best and not slouching. No cell phones, no talking, no resting until you are done for the session. Give it that much intensity and I can tell you from personal experience that any exercise you do will give you results no matter what it is. Let's say you go through the list of exercises and you do exercises in a different order than your used to as one way to make things different? Or you do your usual routine because you love it and then you decide that this exercise machine looks pretty bad to the bone and you want to try it out after your routine? Doing this will keep your body on it's toes and keep you motivated and you will keep improving as long as you keep improving on the exercises.

6.Always focus on improvement

Although this can be lumped with your training journal I want to emphasize this important principle. If it took you 2 hours to do 100 burpees, which of course is an exaggeration, and in one year you could do 100 in 5 minutes, wouldn't your body be fitter, stronger, and better looking? How about if you could only squat 20kg and in one year you were able to squat 100kg? Wouldn't your butt, hips, and legs be much more defined? Focusing on improvement in all exercises comes with the effort you give. Improvement doesn't just have to be adding weight to the bar, it can be adding repetitions to that same weight or doing the total repetitions you usually do in a lesser time for the workout. If you keep track you'll see you'll quite literally always improve. It's a matter of pushing yourself every time you train. Keep doing this and you'll one day walk past a mirror and think to yourself "wow, I'm more defined!". Can't stress enough to not be one of those people that take their shirts off and take pictures in public toilets or gyms. Please take a picture in your own home, and throw a banana peel at the rest of the community that does do the former...Actually throw them a soy injected white potato.

7.Be persistent and be patient

I don't care if someone offers you results by the time the clock strikes midnight and you'll all of a sudden be awarded flowers, a tiara, and the title of ms.world. Or if you were a guy, you'd have a 20-pack, muscles on your muscles, muscles on your eyes, and a money bed with two beautiful women. It isn't going to happen and if someone promises such miracles it's obviously too good to be true. No one is going to lose 100 pounds of fat a night and if it were to happen think of how the health consequences will effect you or think how long you would actually be able to sustain such an appearance. If you want permanent results, and a lifestyle that you have to be happy with, you have to make your body adapt to that lifestyle and you have to work for your body to adapt to it. All good things that are worth something take time and work. Every workout you do, every day you are active, and every day that you eat well, will be a quantum leap forward to your goals. Just when you think you will fail, you are improving.

8. Train a minimum of 10-30 minutes a day

To the clever people who love to say they have done something, and that something was 2 push-ups, this guideline is for you. I want you to do 10 minutes as a bare minimum of hard work and 30 minutes if you weren't feeling your oats (or should I say feeling your steak), because you were very sore from the last legendary workout you did. 10 minutes, when done right, with all your effort, is a mission and will derive all of the benefits you seek due to the amount of work you push yourself to do and 30 minutes is a reasonable amount to get you sweating and active when you do some light activity such as swimming, the best you can, the day after you push yourself beyond your limits. Remember, these are minimums. If you feel like you want to do more, you can.

Warming up

If you have time and when you can help it you have to warm up before you start going all out. A warm-up should be 5-10 minutes. If you are doing weight training, no excuses! Warm up! A simple 5 minute jog, skipping, or star jumps will suffice. The next 5 minutes should consist of loosening up your joints so do some shoulder circles, kick your legs up one at a time, circle your wrists, ankles and knees. If it is especially cold on the day you train then I suggest you warm up 10 minutes with the jump rope, jog or star jumps. In fact, this might be all you need. The reason why this is important is because it gets your body ready with synovial fluid which helps protect you from injury. When your body knows it is ready to train, you'll know by feeling warm and feeling loosened up instead of stiff and cold. As an aside, do NOT static stretch before you train. Your muscles, when you exercise are supposed to contract, which means to shorten. When you static stretch, your muscles are supposed to lengthen. What this means is it can resort to injuries and in some cases can even lead to a lost of strength in some movements (not permanently, but just for the session).

The five ways to train

So now you have the philosophy of training down and how to warm up it's time to talk about the five ways to train.

First: Timed challenge

Get a kitchen timer, a stopwatch, an application on the smart phone for an interval timer or get a gym boss interval timer. Set the time for 1-3 exercises and do them till the time is up. An example can be doing burpees for 10 minutes, doing squats for five minutes, doing squats for 2 minutes, push ups for 2 minutes, burpees for 2 minutes. The list is endless.

Second: Distance challenge

Set down some cones, or just use a landmark such as a tree, and do an exercise until you have reached that distance, and if you want, go back to the start. An example can be dumbbell lunges for 500 yards or bear crawls for a football field. Just tailor it to your difficultly level and try cover more and more distance each time you train.

Third: Repetition challenge

Set a total number of repetitions to complete. An example can be doing 100 total push ups and 100 total mountain jumpers. You don't have to just get to 100 for the push ups before you move on to the mountain jumpers either! You can do as many push ups as you can then do as many jumpers as you can and repeat until you get 100 for each.

Fourth: Rounds challenge

Pick 2-3 exercises and either put a number on the repetitions of the exercises or put a time limit on each and go through each exercise then rest and repeat until you get to the certain number of rounds you do. Let's say you decide to do 7 rounds of sprints, dips, and chin-ups. For a timed tag on these exercises you will do 30 seconds of each exercise (30 second sprints, 30 seconds dips and 30 seconds chin ups) then you will rest for 30 seconds-1 minute and repeat until you have done 7 rounds. For a repetition tag on each exercise you can do 10 yard sprints 10 dips 10 chin ups for the 7 rounds with 30 seconds to one minute of rest in between. Just keep in mind that you will want to keep the rests for each round 1 minute max. Any more than that and you're slacking. If you cannot do 10 repetitions for an exercise because that was the number you gave it, you simply go to the next exercise. So as an example let's say you nailed the sprints but instead of being able to do 10 push ups like you did the last 4 rounds you only got 6, you move on to chin ups.

Fifth: Combined challenge

Just like this sounds, you can combine all the above challenges into one session. You can do lunges with dumbbells for distance, squats for 100 repetitions and you can do burpees for 1 minute for 5 rounds. Create a workout for yourself and challenge yourself in the most fun and interesting fashion. Maybe you like to do a certain exercise for repetitions and another for time, another for distance and maybe you like to do rounds because it gives you an aim. It's all up to you! Be creative!

As a final note with making your own training up, everyone starts somewhere. You go at your own pace with the workouts and you work as hard as YOU can not as hard as someone else at a different level. Maybe all you can do is five repetitions for five rounds right now and it takes you a full minute to rest in between. Or maybe when doing a timed challenge you can only get fifty repetitions of an exercise for five minutes and you had to take quite a few breathers before you attempted to keep doing your repetitions. It's fine! Just do what you can, the best you can. You keep consistent, and you WILL get better, work much longer, tire less easier, get stronger and in turn get the body you want! Remember, improvement is the name of the game!

If I HAD to...Paleo alternatives

I can appreciate that people have a lifestyle in where they do want to have some of the foods or things still incorporated in their life like having alcohol for an example. If one were to cut out every little pleasure that they look forward to completely then it's not going to take a mad time traveling scientist to figure out that they will eventually resort back to their old ways. So this section is for all the people who just HAVE to have that one little thing still in their life.

If you HAD to drink alcohol

The first thing we have to know is what happens when we drink alcohol in order to understand how to still incorporate this into your life whilst losing fat, keeping it off, and being happy.

First the bad news. Alcohol, when ingested, is converted into substance by the liver called acetate. When you ingest alcohol, the alcohol is what is now being used for energy until it is out of your system. This means your carbohydrates and fats will not be used for all your energy requirements. Not only that but alcohol can be a pain with you craving more carbohydrate type foods. If you ever have a good night out drinking and then a few hours later you feel like you want a pizza or something starchy, then alcohol is a good answer as to why that is (33). Lastly, alcohol is a diuretic. This means that it will dehydrate you.

Want some good news? Alcohol actually can be beneficial in ways. As mentioned before, the alcohol red wine can have cardiovascular benefits (5,6), also can reduce appetite if done right, "Long-term alcohol intake can decrease the total amount of food consumed when food is freely available and the alcoholic individual is often held accountable for their irregular eating behavior." (33). Alcohol can actually improve insulin sensitivity which means that it could help with diabetics and non-diabetics alike by better glycemic control (34). Alcohol can actually increase testosterone levels which means that, although you might not be burning off fat, you will be building muscle if you ingest alcohol after your workout, in fact "significantly for 140-300 min post exercise" (35). Finally alcohol has a pretty significant thermic effect, meaning it takes a bit of energy to digest. So alcohol, while it is commonly accepted that it is roughly 7 calories, it is actually 5.7 calories.

The question now is how do you still have a good time out in that special occasion having a drink, gain all the benefits of alcohol whilst negating the negative effects? First is choosing your alcohol, second is when to take it, third is how much to take and fourth is what to eat on the day you decide to drink.

Choosing your alcohol

Wine would be the best choice, after that would be beers, and finally all the other liquor. The reason being is that wine, we already know does offer cardiovascular benefits, but it also has the least amount of calories. Beer comes 2nd with the least amount of calories and finally the other types of liquor confer the most calories. You just have to bear (beer) in mind that you can still have the other liquors available but you just have to keep a much closer eye on your intake of them.

When to drink up and live it up

We already know that alcohol can improve the glycemic control but in turn can increase your appetite. We also know that alcohol can actually improve testosterone levels in modest amounts. So the solution to help control appetite would be to drink your alcohol with your food. Drinking with your meal not only helps keep the appetite down, but it can also improve your food being ingested, and with the added effect of alcohol taking quite a bit of energy to digest, the food along with it means that your metabolism will be raised at least for a little while. We know that ingestion of alcohol after a workout will increase testosterone too so it makes sense to try and have a workout at least a good hour or so before you decide to go drink.

How much to drink and how frequently

I know that from looking at the benefits of alcohol intake you may think that it might be a good idea to just go crazy, binge, and drink every day. After all, a good boost in testosterone means results for muscle and in turn that means a better body too. Unfortunately it doesn't work that way. Alcohol does have benefits but only if you drink moderately and drink once in awhile. An example is that if you drink 30-40g of alcoholic beverage a day, which is the equivalent to roughly 3 beers or 15 ounces of wine your testosterone can drop. In fact it can drop by as much as 7% at the 3 week mark of continual drinking (37). Binge drinking on the night you decide to go and finally have the good stuff is equally bad. A study shows that 1.5kg of alcohol per gram of bodyweight (which is an insane amount), had their testosterone levels drop by 23%. It even made their cortisol levels elevated by as much as 36%! Cortisol is a stress hormone in our body that breaks down muscle and that stores fat. How long did it take for these dazzling negative effects to occur? 10-16 hours! (38). How about post workout? Wouldn't that negate the effects of binge drinking if you drank immediately after? As mentioned, drinking after a workout can have good effects if the drinking is reasonable, but it will have deleterious effects if you go overboard. Your testosterone WILL go down if you decide to binge drink after a workout to the same point that you'll binge drink at any other time. That means your hard work for fat loss or even muscle gain will actually be almost for nothing (39). So how much is a reasonable amount? 60-70grams of alcohol is a good and there isn't any affect on testosterone significantly decreasing when drinking after training (40). Of course in knowing this, you will still have to calculate roughly how much alcohol is good enough to drink in terms of how many calories you are intaking also. So bottom line? Don't drink too frequently and don't binge drink! Drinking 60-70 grams of alcohol for the night that you do won't be severe.

What to eat on the day that you decide to drink

The last thing that needs to be considered will be your eating plan on the day that you decide to drink. The best plan I can give is to limit your carbohydrate consumption because of the fact that the alcohol intake will make you want to have some, to decrease your fat intake, because the alcohol will impair your body's ability to metabolize fat freely since the alcohol also is now what your body is going to be using for it's energy needs for your activity for the dance floor or whatever shenanigan you decide to get up to that night, and to focus on protein since protein is much more satisfying in terms of controlling your appetite and it has a huge thermic effect (it takes a lot more energy to digest) so you're getting the double whammy of increasing your metabolism. What you should focus on eating this day is lean meats and vegetables. When you do decide to go out and drink, if you can help it, then go somewhere where you can eat mostly meat and vegetables. If you cannot then just remember the rule to eat protein first, carbohydrates 2nd and please control how much you intake. Use your portion control. When you do this you'll be able to get the benefit that the alcohol is being used for your energy source (and since carbohydrates and fats aren't going to be used for your energy source and alcohol is, they'll be stored as fat), you'll still be getting your daily needs with your proteins and vegetables, and you can be a bit more lenient with the drinking since lean meats are lesser in calories than the fatty meat (albeit it has less nutrients than fatty meat but the vegetables times infinity is going to at least take care of a few things), and thus still have a great time in the occasion you do drink and you'll burn fat the next day.

30-DAY PALEO HABIT SIX
<u>Liquids are food too!</u>

For these 30 days you will LIMIT alcohol by keeping an eye on how much you are drinking and not going overboard.

REASON FOR HABIT: We now know how to derive benefits out of alcoholic substances and how to negate the negative effects of it. It is easy to go overboard due to peer pressure and temptation with drinks lying around and the "oh why not" mentality. You can still drink and have a good time but let's put into practice the limit and timing of alcohol. Remember, this is for your results!

If you HAD to eat grains

We already established at length why you shouldn't intake grains if you can avoid it in the first place for health reasons and for fat loss reasons. Grains are much better than that fast food place you are going to anyway and if you had a choice of either eating the grains or the food at that place or you just wanted to keep at least some because it makes your life great in ways that are only explained with unicorns jumping over the moon, then yes there is options! Like all things, you have to remember your food intake is most important so don't be slack and count how many calories are ingested in a serve of grains.

When you go to the store it is best to avoid most of the cereals that are on the shelf because they are loaded with ingredients that will wreck havoc on your body. For diabetics you also want to be aware of how these foods will affect you too since all grains are starchy and are high in carbohydrates. While I am full aware that in grains they have fiber, it is best that if you are diabetic to be aware of something called the glycemic index in food and choose carefully with what you pick in terms of grains. If you are not diabetic you still should be careful too! All grains aren't created equal!

As an example, did you know that there are a variety of different oatmeal? There is instant, rolled, steel oats and oat groats. There might be more but for the sake of the point I am trying to make we'll stick with these. Instant oats are usually the ones that are, well, instant. You microwave them and BAM you have oats! Rolled oats are a little more less processed than the instant oats but still has less nutrients in them compared to steel cut oats and oat groats. In fact it has significantly less fat than their other counter-parts, steel cut and oat groats. It's a shock to some that oatmeal actually does contain omega-3s! Steel cut oats are much more minimally processed and they have many more nutrients in-tact. The best type of oats are oat groats. These are the oats that have omega-3s, much more phosphorus, protein and fiber. The instant oats and the rolled oats are actually quite high in the glycemic index and that means that you will get your insulin levels spiked up quite a bit, which means that you'll have a sugar rush and crash and then you'll feel tired after 2 hours or so.

One more example is rice. I know that a few of you have tradition and it is part of your culture to have your cultural food and it really can't be helped in some cases. There is white rice, brown rice, and black rice. The best rice out of these is black rice since it offers more nutrients than it's other counterparts. So if you were to try and choose rice the best one is the black rice.

So the take home message when it comes to grains is you should be wary of the least minimally processed grains and you should have only the grain that has the most nutritional benefits to you rather than it's counter-parts. Of course you should want to limit it as much as you can and stick with food that has much more benefit to you but alas, I'm not you, and I know that you would want to keep at least some food in your diet plan for whatever reason, and I rather you have something that still has benefit rather than something that has practically no benefit and it's common sense how bad it will be for you.

I still want to eat grains but what about the gluten formed in grains? I want to avoid that. Is there any possible way to have a grain without the gluten?

The answer is YES you actually can have a few grains that don't have the gluten in them. Personally, I love oat groats. Oats actually don't have gluten and not only that but if you were to eat oats and you were known to be hypertensive, it can actually help you out! In a study it helped 72% of the controlled group of people to reduce their anti-hypertensive medication and in turn help with their blood pressure control (42). If grains are also fermented they should be able to remove the gluten content too. Preparation with fermentation is a lot to some people, but if you were that concerned with your health and wanted to still have something that you just can't live without then it has to be done.

If you HAD to eat legumes

Legumes should be avoided period. We already explained why but as a little recap, although foods do have some traces of lecithins and some of phytates, legumes are the superstars of these! Phytates block nutrient absorption and lecithins on the other hand can do a few things, but in particular did you know that lecithin can lessen the mucous in your intestines? (41). If your intestines don't have mucous, that can mean you'll have a host of problems of intestinal inflammation and it might even cause some diseases!

If you still MUST insist on having legumes the best option is to soak the beans in clean, fresh water for a good period of 24 hours and boil it good. Doing this will remove most of the lecithins and phytates. Just keep in mind there will still be traces of these and you should strive to eat less of these if possible.

If you HAD to eat starches

Just like we covered in the grains, you should choose the best option and you should eat starches as a treat more than anything (unless of course you were a pro-athlete). White potato versus a sweet potato? Sweet potato will win since it has more nutritional benefit than a white potato. Getting the best of nutritional benefits from your starches is the first thing you should do. When you eat them just remember to have them last in your meals. Remember you do not want to over-eat and you want to keep in control how much you are intaking. There shouldn't be too much problems

otherwise.

What should you do if...Keeping on track with the plan

The final consideration when getting your results is what to do when you are forced into situations that it seems that you must deviate a little. Can you still go on that trip and come back looking better? What should you do when you have someone hounding you to eat something you know is bad for you and you just plain don't want to eat it? This is what we will tackle now.

What should you do if you don't have enough time to prepare your food for the day?

When you know the next day is going to be busy the first thing you should consider is making your meals in advance. Nothing can make someone go off the rails faster than not having their meal ready and then seeing a fast food place thinking it's a good idea to visit. Tupperware should come in handy for these situations. Simply cook the meals you know you need in advance because you can't cook it on the day and freeze it, thaw it out the next day and nuke it up in the microwave. For you die-hard paleo advocates out there, I realize a microwave doesn't exist in the stone-age times but to all the guys and girls who cannot bare a cold tasting meal then the microwave will come in handy.

Alternatively what you can do is cook a week's worth or half a week's worth of food in one day, freeze the food and thaw whatever you need for whatever day it is you need it. You can also use a slow-cooker if you are stuck for time preparing something yourself by just putting the ingredients in the slow-cooker, setting it on, and when you come home or wake up in the morning your food will be cooked!

If you are still having trouble eating a certain meal that requires preparation at a certain time like lunch then you can either change the meal you thought of with another easy to make meal, or you can swap that meal with another meal you were going to eat that didn't take much preparation. The last alternative is, if you can bare it, just to not eat when you are very busy and eat when you are able to. So if you are busy the whole day with work because you are flying to another place, doing work there and coming back at night time, then why not eat a nice big breakfast and then eat a nice big meal when you get home instead of having the usual lunch?

What if you were pressured to eat/drink for a social situation and didn't want to?

This is going to sound very obvious but this gets to a lot of people. You have to learn to say NO. If the person is still insisting after multiple uses of the greatest word there is in every language, and even insults you, then doesn't it make sense that the person isn't your friend? I don't know or can't say why they would go so far to keep forcing you...Maybe it's the fact that they're insecure? That they want to bring you down to their level? That they are envious? Feel threatened? Or maybe they're just a giant pile of all things that people hate? Whatever the reason, you just say no and walk away. If it was in a family setting and they were forcing you to eat a bunch of cake and someone injected the cake with steroids (and no I've never seen it happen), same thing! Say no! What if you'll hurt their feelings? They're hurting yours right now just by pissing you off, and even your health! That's no respect now is it? If someone likes playing video games in his or her spare time, and you think it's a waste of time, would you insult the person and force the person to stop playing video games? (Note, I said spare time, spare being 2 hours a day tops, not 20 hours a day). How about if that person were to force you to play the video game that they're playing to the point of insulting you after you've said no? If the person plays the video game and respects that you don't want to play, and you, yourself respected that they want to play, then great! I know video games are a weak comparisons to food but hopefully you catch what I'm trying to say. For you hardcore paleos, the game was a caveman game where you have a club, you level up your character while he tackles the harshest barren wastelands and beating up monsters such as the dreaded soy-potato tree. So don't hate mail me that video games aren't paleo.

What should you do if you wanted to have dairy?

As mentioned in this book, it's not bad to have dairy in moderate amounts. What is bad about having dairy is the source you get it from. If you were to get dairy in the supermarket loaded with ingredients then that's not a good idea. Getting milk from the store knowing what UHT, pasteurized, and homogenized means is not a good idea either. In fact getting any product that lists ingredients (which almost all have) that has any type of pasteurized milk isn't too bright. To top it off you'll have concerns about having dairy products that might come from cattle that is laden with hormones. Yogurt in the store isn't going to help either since it's processed and being shipped to the store and now on the shelf in the frozen section you see it in, most of, if not all, the beneficial bacteria you believe will help with your gut bacteria is dead. So what to do?

The best thing you can do is first of all make sure the dairy products are organic and come from grass-fed animals. That will mean you'll have to go to an organic store or farmer's market and ask a farmer at one of the stalls about it.

Usually organic shops have the quality you are after and all the cattle used to make the dairy are free-roaming and grass-fed all their life. If you want to take it a step further, you can ring the farmer themselves and ask about the conditions. For the ultra-paranoid, you can go visit their farm.

Milk should be raw but if you were to have it raw it should come from sources that are well looked after, clean, and the milk should be consumed immediately. Not only that but make sure that it is coming from grass-fed cows and they are not injected with hormones. I advise raw milk because it has the enzyme that other milk lacks, lactase, which is needed to digest milk, and all the minerals and vitamins are intact. If you still insist in having pasteurized milk, seeing as it's the better option, just make sure you have it fresh and the source is good. Ideally you could try get the raw milk yourself and boil it yourself and thus pasteurizing yourself knowing that you didn't put anything else in there or heated it to the utmost amount. You cannot purchase raw milk legally from stores so my best bet would be to own a share of a cow from a farmer local to you.

Whey is a dairy product and you would definitely have heard of it from all the supplements out there. Whey is essentially the protein powder you all hear. Whey is also a derived by cheese. So when you eat cheese, that is also whey. If you were to have this, I would advise not buying the whey from the supplement shops that are loaded with ingredients. What you are after is just the whey itself. It doesn't exactly matter if it is whey concentrate or isolate, just get something that the only ingredient in there is whey. Some health shops and supplement stores might have it, but your best bet again would be to go to an organic shop.

What should you do if you were on the road or on vacation?

Let's say you were planning a road trip to somewhere or your job entails that you are on the road all the time. Prepare your meals in advance. The tupperware tip helps here. If you like your food warm I would advise you to invest in a slow cooker put the food on low before you go to sleep, this way when you wake up you'll have a readily warm meal and you can put the food in your tupperware.

If you were on vacation this isn't an excuse to not have a choice, because there ALWAYS is a choice! Going to a restaurant that serves steak or any other type of meat is an option. It wouldn't be too hard to find a steak-house if you were in the city would it? Or how about a seafood restaurant? If you were that dedicated you could visit a grocery store and buy yourself some tuna in a can or chicken. While I don't advise one eat this on a daily basis since there is mercury on the cans, if you look at the ingredients to be sure that there isn't any harmful substances you'll be alright. You can make your own little salad dish just by buying a bed of greens, some tuna and chicken in the can (and be sure to drain out the spring water), some nuts and apple cider vinegar along with some fruit. If you like it spicy you can add tabasco sauce. You can do this if you are stuck somewhere where there isn't a good option in the meantime until a few hours later where you find yourself a better option if this is the case.

If you are in the hotel you could even ask the chef for specific orders on your foods. In one hotel I visited there wasn't a beef omelet on the menu so I asked if it was possible to make a beef and vegetable omelet. There was salads that had sauces I didn't agree with so I simply asked for the salad but with no sauces. This tip doesn't just have to be at hotels either, it can be used in restaurants too.

What should you do if you wanted to have something sweet

I can understand that most people would have a craving for something sweet, this seems to be the most asked. Let me tell you that first of all, you are probably addicted if you can't even go 1 week without having a withdrawal or thinking about having something sweet constantly. My best advice is to get rid of this craving first. 2-3 weeks is usually enough time for someone to best this craving.

You'll find that when you give up all those really concentrated sweets that you find in abundance in such things as that cake you had or that chocolate you got at the store that even fruit tastes sweet enough! Fruit is allowed on this plan, it is beneficial, and this should be more than enough for your sweet tooth. If this still fails then my 2nd advice, while it isn't considered paleo, is to mix in some RAW honey with your food. I can't stress enough that the honey should be raw. Honey in the store has a lot of bad ingredients in it such as high fructose corn syrup as mentioned in the ingredients section. The honey is also heated so it's shelf life can last longer. Raw honey on the other hand has some beneficial assets. It can provide nitric oxide, (mead, which is honey and red wine, is used in the honeymoon as old tradition by the vikings to make one more fertile), and can potentially help the immune system. Honey has been used as a cure for wounds in the past also. My only gripe with honey is that it's almost like pure sugar and it's fructose levels are quite high. You can over-do the honey by adding massive spoon-fulls to whatever you mix it with. If you insist in having honey only add a small amount. A tablespoon would be more than enough to make any serving sweet, and that, in itself, is actually the good news! So substitute your sugar uses with RAW honey and you'll still enjoy a little sweet in your life. As for me, no thanks, I'm sweet enough.

If you HAD to take a day off training

EVERYONE and I mean EVERYONE has at least 10 minutes to spare in their day. There is NO excuses! NONE! If you are injured? Then work a body part that isn't injured. Example can be if you broke both legs and broke both your wrists and broke your back all at once, and thus being bed-ridden, guess what you can do? Move your arms up and down as many times as you can, cross them over your chest and back out as many times as you can, lift your knees toward your chest (if able) and back down. Work your neck. Whatever! Do something! Kegels!

Training every day, as mentioned, doesn't mean you have to go hard every single day. Maybe there will be days where you aren't injured physically but you are injured emotionally? Maybe you lost someone dear to you and, unless you were like me, training is the last thing you want to do. Believe it or not, training still helps. Going hardcore when you are emotionally stressed will probably only benefit someone who is naturally inclined to take it all out on something, that something being themselves, or it's just something that makes them happy, that they love. In these situations, a walk outside by yourself with some headphones on at a fast pace to music still helps and still constitutes as training doesn't it? Going for a swim or riding a bike out to some place you like? Yep, training.

The last excuse I hear is, what if I'm on a plane, or in a car all day? If you are in a car, then pull over and just do it! If you are on a plane, sure you can be me, and do push ups in the isles till you get told you're an idiot and asked to sit back down, then secretly go to the toilet and do squats for an hour while people start knocking saying that they need to pee and they think that you're probably masturbating, and so you use that as the reason it took you so long so the flight sheriff doesn't tie you up to your chair so you can't do anything....yes real experience. Anyway. What you can do instead is do calf raises on your seat, flex your muscles as hard as possible or do some "imaginary weights training" by pitting one muscle against the other. Things like putting your right hand on your left hand or wrist and using your left arm to do a bicep curl while the right arm being "the weight". This was a method of training by someone named Charles Atlas back in the times of the golden age of strongmen and one of the rumors is (which it isn't true) he discovered this way of exercising by going to the zoo and seeing how lions keep in shape. How paleo does that get?

The point is, you can do something, anything, every day. No sleep and body's super fatigued? Go walk or swim. Take it easy. Feel great and just got off the plane and now in the hotel? Go for it!

CLIFF NOTES FOR THE CONFUSED AND IMPATIENT

CHAPTER FOUR

1. Mindset: The mindset is the most important thing for results. Whatever training you decide to do you have to give it your all and you have to constantly improve. No slacking!

2. Training philosophy:

Train everyday

Train 10-30 minutes at a time

Do as much as you can do in a certain time frame in the session

Keep a log book of your training

Do exercises that work the whole body and not just one part of the body

Always do something different

Always focus on improvement

Be persistent and patient

3. The five ways to train:

Time based: Pick an amount of time for an exercise and go for it. E.G. 10 minutes of burpees

Distance based: Cover a certain distance E.G. Bear Crawl 250 yards

Repetition based: Pick a total amount of repetitions E.G. 100 burpees

Rounds based: Finish a certain number of rounds E.G. 15 rounds of 15 second sprints with 30 seconds of rest

Combined: Any of the four mentioned training combined to your liking

Don't forget to warm up with 5 minutes of jogging, star jumps or skipping. Don't static stretch before you train.

4. If you had to drink alcohol: Wines are the best choice, beer comes 2nd and other liquor comes 3rd. If you were to drink alcohol be sure not to go over-board with your drinking and not drink every single day. Alcohol converts into acetate and will be your energy source when drinking so be sure to limit carbohydrates and fats on the day you are drinking and stick to lean meat and vegetables. Drink with your meal and have a workout an hour or so before you decide to drink.

5. If you had to eat grains: Oatmeal (oat groats and steel cuts are the best. Avoid instant oats) are fine as well as fermented grains since they don't contain traces of gluten. Since they are starchy however be sure you are always active when eating these.

6. If you had to eat starches: Choose the better option E.G. Sweet potatoes are better than white potatoes. Eat starches on your most active days and preferably after you train.

7. If you had to eat legumes: Best advice is not to but if you did have to, you would be best to soak them at least 24 hours and boil them good.

8. If you had to have dairy: Check the source and make sure they are good

9. What should you do if you didn't have time to prepare food the next day?: Cook food in advance. Put them in tupperware and freeze it, thaw it out when needed and heat it in the microwave. You can also invest in a slow-cooker.

10. What should you do if you were pressured in a situation where you were forced to eat and drink things you didn't want to?: Say no and walk away.

11. What should you do if you were on the road or vacation: Cook meals in advance, check grocery stores, ask the chef at hotel to modify orders, find restaurants that serve good food.

12. What should you do if you wanted something sweet: Add raw honey to some of your meals and eat fruit.

13. What should you do if you had to take a day off training: You don't. You can be active for 10 minutes a day anyway possible. No excuses.

14. Habit six: Limit your drinking. Don't go over-board with it. Learn to say no and learn to control yourself in social situations.

Chapter five: Tricks and tips to burn that fat

"Chuck Norris destroyed the periodic table because Chuck Norris only recognizes the element of surprise" -Chucknorrisfacts.com

What plan wouldn't be complete with the extra tools to enable you to truly lose all the fat you want? Body isn't agreeing with you to lose fat? Then it's time to implement a few strategies to send those adipose tissues straight to the center of the earth! Here's a few tips that might be beneficial for you.

Tip three: Ketogenic dieting

Let's use good ol' wikipedia to describe what ketogenic dieting is:

"The ketogenic diet is a high-fat, adequate-protein, low-carbohydrate diet that in medicine is used primarily to treat difficult-to-control epilepsy in children. The diet forces the body to burn fats rather than carbohydrates" (45).

This is useful in a few ways. The first being useful to fight off sugar cravings that most have. If you ever have gone off having no carbohydrates and none of those concentrated sweets for a period of two weeks then you introduced fruit back into your body I can attest that you WILL be able to taste how much sweeter it is.

Secondly for some people, they thrive off this lifestyle. Maybe some actually don't have a taste for sweets as mentioned throughout the book but are still stuck in their ways with processed meat and their other problem is starches. We all know that anything that's processed is bad, and to top that off, if you're one of the many who get flavored enhanced this or that then this will make the transition easier.

The third is that it can help with is the control of weight, blood glucose concentrations for diabetics, hunger, diet satisfaction and it can help keep your energy levels stable. All this despite you having to drop calories. This means that instead of feeling like you're out of energy due to cutting food and feeling like you are still hungry after a meal, a ketogenic diet, with carbohydrates as low as 20grams a day, you will still feel good and feel like you had a decent meal (46).

Another benefit is that ketogenic dieting has been shown to help with people who suffer epilepsy. (48) Also, adding MCT oils (medium chain triglyceride oils), helps with people who suffer from this condition (49).

You would naturally have to cut calories in order to lose fat and doing a ketogenic diet at the beginning would be best to control your sugar and hunger cravings. Not only that, but when you do decide to have a little carbohydrate or sweet treat, due to the insulin sensitivity you gain from this, you'll be able to better tolerate it, and least likely to put on fat since you need to replenish your glycogen stores from the carbohydrates (46).

If you are coming from an obese background then a ketogenic diet can kick start you the right way in terms of fat loss. If you have a lot of fat to lose, the ketogenic diet shows that it can lower your bad LDL cholesterol, increase your good HDL cholesterol, it can also significantly reduce your triglycerides (the fat you are trying to get rid of). If you decide to follow this way of eating long-term until you get lean, there are no ill-effects (47). Since you already have enough triglycerides to burn, and that means, you have much more stored energy to use, enabling your body to use that energy instead of having the energy to be used by outside sources of food (which is your carbohydrates you intake) will mean that you'll have an easier time losing fat at the start. As you get leaner to the point where you do have a six-pack or that hour-glass figure, then your body will be able to better tolerate carbohydrates more simply because you do not have that reserve energy anymore since you burned it off your body. Remember, the adipose tissue you carry is stored energy, and your goal with exercise and cutting food intake is to let your body use that energy. To let the body rely on it's fat stores means that this is a powerful method in reducing body fat.

Ketogenic dieting also can be used as a tool for sustainable fat loss. When you know you will pig out the next day due to an occasion and will have a few carbohydrates, you can simply use ketogenic dieting for the days leading up to that occasion so you can increase your insulin sensitivity to better use the carbohydrates rather than store them. Think of ketogenic dieting like a sandbox if you will. When you deplete your muscles and body of carbohydrates via ketogenic dieting you are taking sand out of the sandbox (the sand being carbohydrates) and when you have too many carbohydrates your sandbox gets filled beyond what it is capable, leaving you with a mess to clean up (which means fat). An example of how effective ketogenic dieting really is in terms of fat loss is a recent study that shows a group of people who adhered to a ketogenic diet and a Mediterranean diet. They would switch back and forth between the two every 2 weeks or so, and with the Mediterranean diet being the one consumed the last 6 months of the study. Every time the group switched to ketogenic dieting, they lost significant fat (50).

How to use ketogenic dieting effectively

From the information we gathered above, to use ketogenic dieting you first need to limit your carbohydrates to less than 30g a day. Best time to take carbohydrates would be after you train since your muscles are depleted as it is and it would help them shuttle nutrients into your muscle. If you have a lot of fat to lose (for men that is over 25 percent body fat and for women, over 35 percent) you can use ketogenic dieting from the beginning and you can continue to use it until you are on the average side of body fat percentiles (for men that would be 15-18% and for women roughly 20-25 percent). When you are on the average percentiles you can now add carbohydrates back in and this is where if you were to go out and socialize and eat some carbohydrate type foods you can do so. Doing this will actually give your body a break from the ketogenic dieting as well as a mental one too and this will be explained by the next weight loss trick.

Tip two: Overfeeding to lose fat

Yes, you can actually have a point where you can over-eat to enable you to lose fat further, and this method is a tool to actually help you get over your fat loss plateau when you come to the point where you are having consistent weight loss for months, but then you find yourself not losing it and need a break. The popular term of this is called "cheat meals", and the reason why it is called so is because a day such as this will allow you to eat foods that are forbidden. I'm not an a fan of saying when you have these over feedings you should strive to eat a pizza to the maximum since after all there are much better choices to get nutrients from your foods out there, but what this method can also do for you is, when you are planning to go and celebrate a social occasion, such as a wedding, Christmas holidays or even a date, then this will come in handy too. The purpose of this method physiologically is to make your body be tricked into thinking you are overfed and that there isn't any sense of a famine (which is one of the reasons after consistent weight loss, your body will catch on and not want to lose fat) and therefore your body is more willing to burn more fat.

The science behind overfeeding

When you overfeed from a period of low calorie dieting for a certain time the body will catch on as mentioned. There is a hormone in the body that is responsible for our hunger levels and to be aware if we are actually in a famine. You have to ask yourself, how is it that our body knows when food must become available and how does it exactly know to conserve energy to protect our vital organs and functions from harm? The answer is this hormone called **leptin.**

"Leptin is an adipocyte-secreted hormone that regulates appetite and energy balance of the body and has an important role in adaptation during underfeeding and overfeeding. It takes a significant task in controlling hypothalamic-pituitary growth, adrenal and gonadal functions." (51)

From that quote you can see that it is the very hormone that tells us to hold on to our fat stores and to be more hungry when needed, and it has a role to tell the anabolic hormones in our body to grow and sex hormones that it is fine to be produced. Control this hormone you and can control your fat loss. This hormone can very well be the answer to why you are not losing fat when you are getting to the stages where you are getting lean. The reason why it is not a good idea to overeat and use this strategy when you still have a lot of fat to lose is because "leptin are increased in proportion to body fat stores as a result of increased production in enlarged fat cells from obese subjects" (54). So the leaner you are, the more beneficial this will work and the more frequently you can use this, while the more fat you have, the less you are able to use it. You must earn your right to eat treat yourself first.

To sum up, what are the benefits an overfeeding meal?

Overfeeding can be shown to increase the response from your adrenal glands and replenish your sex hormones plus speed up your metabolism (speed up metabolism if the meal was a mix of carbohydrates and fats and if you did not have much fat to spare) (52).

How to use overfeeding meals effectively

Overfeeding is best done after a period where you focus on losing weight and when you restrict yourself from carbohydrates. The reason why it is good to restrict carbohydrates leading up to when you decide to overeat is because when you do overeat and you have your abundance of carbohydrates from foods that aren't considered paleo, carbohydrates have a more significant effect on increasing leptin (in overfeeding with carbohydrates alone "increased plasma leptin concentrations by 28%") while fat does not (in overfeeding with fat alone "did not significantly change plasma leptin concentrations") (53). When overeating you MUST overeat. No holding back. You have to eat your fill. The purpose of this is so your leptin stores are high and your body knows it isn't in a state of starvation and therefore will lose fat when you get back to dieting. It takes roughly 24 hours to get your leptin back to normal levels and it is all from the meal that you eat.

"increases in serum leptin starts to occur approximately 4-7 h after meals. Increasing evidence indicates that insulin, in concert with permissive effects of cortisol, can increase serum leptin over this time frame and likely contributes to meal-induced increases in serum leptin." (54).

Alternatively, if you do not like to have the one big meal you can have a whole day where you can eat forbidden foods. Still not working for you? Then you can take a period of a week or two weeks where you eat over your maintenance of calories and then go back to eating to lose fat by going under your maintenance. I will outline three ways to use this tool.

The overfeeding way one: Planning for that social event (just the one event)

With this way of overfeeding you cut out the carbohydrates for a period of a week at least and keep your calories to how it would be when you are trying to lose weight. The day before you decide to binge you have lean meats instead of fatty meats (like chicken breasts without the skin), along with vegetables. When the day of the event comes, eat like the day before (the lean meats and vegetables) then when it's time for the event, go for it. Have a set period of time where you are allowed to eat whatever you want as much as you want. If it's game night and you are playing poker with your buddies, or for you girls, your girlfriend is getting married and you are having a bachelorette party, that'll usually last quite long, these are perfect scenarios where you can have a five hour period where you allow yourself to eat! To also answer, no, it is advisable not to eat the food off the stripper if it is a guy. If it is a girl however that is fine. You can repeat this cycle every week if you choose to for awhile to take a break (make sure you are lean though! Lean being at least 15% and under body fat for men and under 20% for women!) Here's an outline how it works:

Overfeeding for that one event plan						
DAY 1:	DAY 2:	DAY 3:	DAY 4:	DAY 5:	DAY 6:	DAY 7: (EVENT DAY)
No carbohydrates, only lean meats and vegetables	Ketogenic dieting	Ketogenic dieting	Ketogenic	Ketogenic dieting	No carbohydrates, only lean meats and vegetables	Lean meats for the day, 5 hour period of overeating when event arises

Notes: You can drink alcohol on this day. Drinking will help with insulin sensitivity and since you have depleted your body quite a bit you can be more lenient. Of course, do not go overboard as always. If you want a pizza you can have your pizza or two. If you want to eat clean then make sure that the meal is mixed with fats and carbohydrates with an emphasis on the carbohydrates. That means you can have steak and potatoes with a cake for dessert if you were celebrating a birthday or if you were out on a date to an Asian restaurant you can have more sushi, spring rolls etc. Yes this isn't exactly paleo but this is after all a technique to keep you sane and help you get over the plateau you are having. If you want something paleo-esque you can have your favorite meat and sweet potatoes and pumpkin galore as one example.

The overfeeding way two: the day of chaos

This is like the first one except now it's the whole day. Some people don't like to splurge on just one sitting or a period of hours and some just like to take a day to take a break and find it much easier to eat. If this is the case then nothing has changed with the outline, just the time you eat, which means you start eating this way as soon as the day starts.

The overfeeding way three: one-two week breather

This way is what I would recommend since you can still stick to eating paleo much better, and you can focus on building muscle in the mean time. Not only that, but you can get away with a little treat here and there.

So let's say you hit your plateau and for two months you haven't lost fat. It's time to implement this outline:

Overeating way three: one-two week breather						
Week one and two Day 1: Eat over maintenance by 250-500 calories	Day 2: Same	Day 3: Same	Day 4: Same	Day 5: Same	Day 6: Same	Day 7: Same
NOTES: If you want to include your treat then simply just add the calories of the treat and there you go. I would advise if you are doing two weeks of this to up the						

calories around 250-350 for maintenance and if you are just doing one week to up the calories by 500. If you are interested in taking a longer period of time like 3 weeks then increase the calories to 250.

Week 3: Get back to reducing caloric intake by 500. Pick up where you left off by going back to doing your starting point, planning your meals etc.

Keep one thing in mind when using this method: it is NOT something you do everyday and every weekend for the whole entire year. This is a tool that if sparingly used it is very beneficial. If you were going away on vacation for one month and you wanted to live it up on the weekend every weekend for your whole trip, then you can! Then when you get back home you can readjust and go back to your eating to lose fat and break past your plateau. This is one example. Or if you were just stuck and you now see your 4-pack abdominals and wanted to lose more, then this can help by you working with your body.

To make this even MORE effective, it is best to train before you decide to have your overeating meals, and if you were doing the two weeks of overeating, then of course it is beneficial to train for the 2 weeks. The reason is that the carbohydrates will be more beneficial to be used to your muscles by restoring glycogen since the muscles are depleted from carbohydrates (remember that sandbox analogy?) and negate most effects that could come with the overeating.

You can combine overeating with ketogenic dieting for great results also. The trick is to do ketogenic dieting 6 days in the week (which means no carbohydrates and high fat intake along with medium protein intake) and to have low fat but high carbohydrate intake on the 7th day (which means stuff like cake, pastries etc).

Again, remember, this is a tool to use sparingly. It is a very powerful tool and one designed to lose fat. I personally would recommend to stick to healthier options than a pizza (like oat groats mixed in honey and cocoa butter), or something that can still be paleo-esque (like sweet potatoes and beets), but I understand that you do have those occasions and this is how you can handle those occasions and holidays and come back much more leaner than ever before! Not only that, but this will help you maintain your well-deserved body you have worked hard for in the long run.

Tip three: Eat your carbohydrates at night

This can very well tie in with your overeating methods. I can hear a lot of you now telling me "what the utter fruit? But if I eat carbohydrates at night they won't be used and I'll get fat!" Actually the direct opposite will happen. A study shows that there was two groups of people. One that ate the majority of their carbohydrates during the day and the other that ate their carbohydrates at night. How much was the majority of the carbohydrates consumed at night? 80%! The results? The group that ate carbohydrates at night lost more fat, their insulin sensitivity improved, they felt more satiated and had decreased inflammation! How much fat was lost compared to the other group? 28%! If you still don't believe that it's possible, consider that both groups ate the same amount of calories (55).

There is a common belief that your energy expenditure slows down when you sleep. This is true but it is also true that there are rises and falls when you sleep, such as your energy expenditure increases when you enter a deep sleep state also called REM (56).

One more note just to sell you on the fact that you won't get fat if you have your carbohydrates, and the majority of carbohydrates at night at that. When you exercise, the effect of you training lets you burn fat much more during sleep since it increases the sleeping metabolic rate significantly (57).

So now you can use this tip two ways. When trying to lose weight you can eat the majority of your carbohydrates at night time when you are eating how this book is instructed for you to lose weight. The second is when you are planning to overfeed yourself using the first way to overfeed (overfeeding with a period of 5 hours), by having your period of eating in the early till late evening.

CLIFF NOTES FOR THE CONFUSED AND IMPATIENT

CHAPTER FIVE

1. Ketogenic dieting: Ketogenic dieting is to limit your carbohydrates to below 20g a day so your body can rely on fat stores for fuel instead of carbohydrates. If you have a lot of fat to lose, ketogenic dieting can be a good way to kick start.

2. Overfeeding: When you are getting to the stages where you are getting lean or you hit a plateau because your body discovers that you are losing weight and it thinks you are dying you have to let your body know that you aren't dying by controlling the hormone leptin. By strategically overeating you'll be able to let leptin happy and thus get over your plateau. You can overeat by having a planned event where you can overeat for a 5 hour period, have a whole day, or have 1-2 weeks where you eat

250-500 calories over your maintenance calories. To use this effectively you must limit your carbohydrate intake as well as calories leading up to the overeating period for one week at a MINIMUM. This should only be used when you are at a plateau, a plateau being that you haven't lost any fat at all for 2 months.

3. Eating the majority of your carbohydrates at night: This actually is a good thing. It will help you feel more fuller and it can even help you lose fat!

Chapter six: Five Paleo slow-cooker recipes

"Get in ma belly!" - Fat Bastard character in Austin Powers movie

What nutrition book wouldn't be complete with at least some recipes? The reason I chose slow-cooker recipes to include here is not only because it is one of my favorite methods of cooking, but because it'll help those of you that have the issue of time with preparing your meals. These recipes will contain serving size and nutritional facts such as calories so you don't have to worry about trying to figure out yourself how many protein, carbohydrates or fats each have.

Shameless plug: **If you want more recipes like this then you can go check out my other book: 30 day Paleo diet slow cooker recipe cookbook: Delicious, easy recipes to cook and eat at home that restore health and lose weight. These recipes listed in this book are samples of what to expect.** Alternatively you can visit my website: HTTP://www.paindoesnthurt.com as I post recipes there for FREE from time to time when I'm not posting more nutrition and training info (far beyond the scope of this book).

Now, ahem, with that out of the way! On to the recipes! Please try not to eat this book as I do not know how many calories paper has but I'm sure it isn't going to help you lose fat.

Spicy Brownies

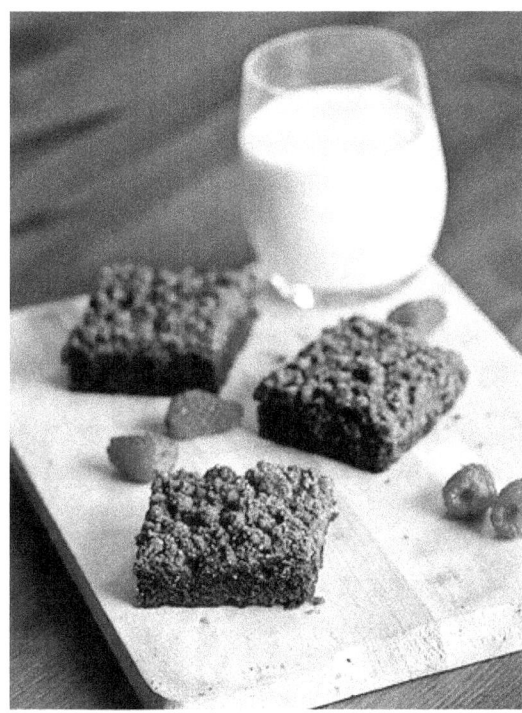

Yes, you read that right – brownies with a heat kick. Chocolate and chili is a combination that lasts for centuries already. Don't worry about the heat though; it's not that strong and definitely not overpowering the taste of the brownies. It just emphasizes the aroma of chocolate and makes it a special dessert.

Prep time: 15 minutes

Cook time: 8 hours

Servings: 8

Ingredients:

1 cup buckwheat flour

¼ cup coconut flour

½ cup cocoa powder

1 pinch salt

¼ teaspoon chili powder

1 teaspoon baking soda

¼ cup raw honey

½ cup coconut oil

4 eggs

Directions:

1. In a bowl, combine the buckwheat flour with the coconut flour, cocoa powder, salt, chili powder and baking soda.

2. In a different bowl, combine the raw honey with the coconut oil and eggs.

3. Mix the dry ingredients with the wet ones and give it a good mix.

4. Pour the batter into your slow cooker and cook on low settings for 8 hours.

5. When done, cut into small squares and serve with a glass of almond milk.

Nutritional information per serving

Calories: 184

Fat: 19.6g

Protein: 5.3g

Carbohydrates: 17.6g

Kale and Mushroom Quiche

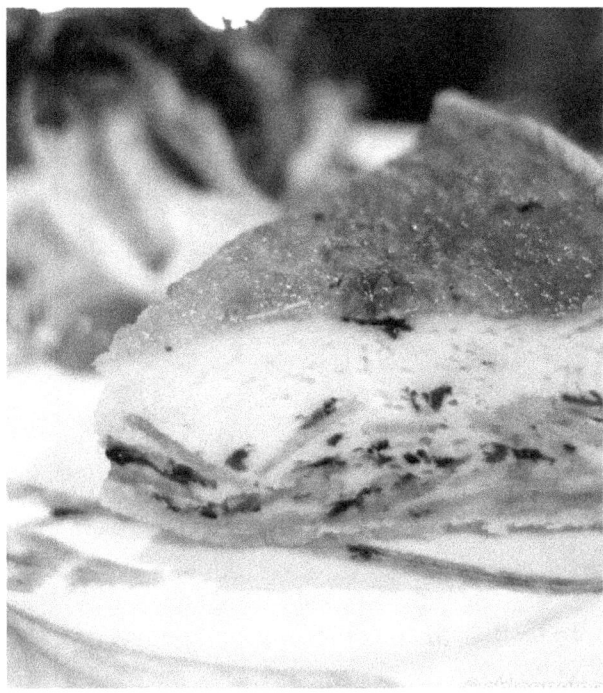

Rich in flavors, this quiche is perfect for your morning meals. Turn the crock pot on the night before to make sure it's ready for breakfast and feel free to customize the recipes by adding more vegetables or replacing the ones found in the recipe.

Prep time: 20 minutes

Cook time: 8 hours

Servings: 8

Ingredients:

8 kale leaves, shredded

1 bacon slice, fat trimmed then chopped

4 Portobello mushrooms, sliced

1 pound champignon mushrooms, sliced

1 red bell pepper, cored and chopped

6 eggs

2 oz. cashew nuts, soaked over night

2 tablespoons chopped parsley

Salt, pepper to taste

Directions:

1. Place the eggs and cashews in a blender and pulse until smooth. Transfer into a large bowl.

2. Stir in the kale and chopped bacon, as well as the mushrooms, bell pepper, parsley, salt and freshly ground pepper.

3. Pour the mixture into your slow cooker. Turn it on and cook for 8 hours on low settings.

4. Serve the quiche warm or cold, with a fresh salad preferably.

Nutritional information per serving

Calories: 99

Fat: 5.3g

Protein: 7.3g

Carbohydrates: 5.5g

Breakfast Zucchini Lasagna

Unlike the typical lasagna, this recipe is not only cooked on a crock pot, but also is lighter and has more vegetables, yielding a flavorful and absolutely delicious breakfast. It uses zucchinis instead of lasagna noodles, but you can replace them with eggplant for a variation of this recipe.

Prep time: 20 minutes

Cook time: 8 hours

Servings: 8

Ingredients:

1 pound mushrooms, finely chopped

2 eggs

¼ teaspoon cayenne pepper

1 teaspoon dried basil

1 teaspoon dried oregano

1 teaspoon cumin powder

2 young zucchinis, finely sliced lengthwise

1 cup cashew nuts, soaked over night

2 tablespoons lemon juice

2 tablespoons fresh dill

2 cups fresh tomato puree

Salt, pepper to taste

Directions:

1. Blend the cashews with the fresh dill, lemon juice, salt and pepper until smooth. Set aside.

2. In a bowl, mix the mushrooms with the eggs, cayenne pepper, basil, oregano, cumin powder, salt and pepper

3. Start layering the zucchini slices, mushrooms, cashew sauce and tomato puree into your crockpot. End with a layer of tomato puree.

4. Bake on low settings for 8 hours and serve the lasagna warm.

Nutritional information per serving

Calories: 143

Fat: 10.6g

Protein: 7g

Carbohydrates: 10.4g

Roasted Red Pepper and Spinach Frittata

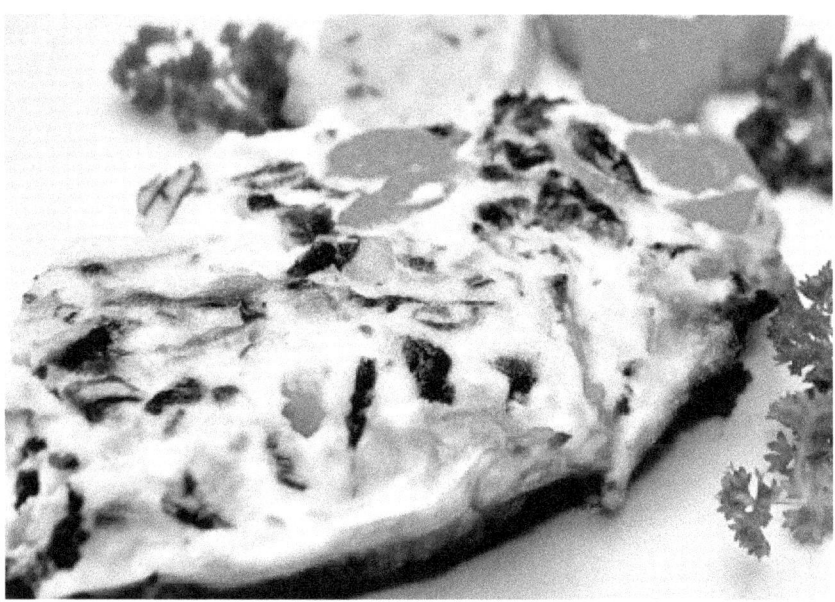

Frittata has Spanish origins and it's very similar to an omelet, but it uses more vegetables, it's creamy and the flavors are more intense unlike omelets which tend to be much simpler, with fewer ingredients, focusing more on the eggs than the additional ingredients.

Prep time: 15 minutes

Cook time: 6 hours

Servings: 6

Ingredients:

6 eggs, beaten

1 sweet potato, peeled and diced

2 cups baby spinach leaves

2 red bell peppers, roasted (canned)

½ cup cherry tomatoes, quartered

1 pinch smoked paprika

1 teaspoon dried basil

Salt, pepper to taste

Directions:

1. Mix all the ingredients in your slow cooker.

2. Cover with its lid and cook on low settings for 6 hours.

3. Serve slightly warm, sliced, topped with a fresh salad if you want or just a few tomato slices.

Nutritional information per serving

Calories: 124

Fat: 4.2g

Protein: 14.8g

Carbohydrates: 12.7g

Aromatic Herbed White Fish

White fish is very mild and doesn't have that strong distinctive taste or aroma that most fish does. For that reason, it can easily be paired with a wide variety of spices and herbs in our case. They infuse the white meat, transforming it into a fragrant dish. Served drizzled with lemon juiced it can be an amazing and light dinner.

Prep time: 15 minutes

Cook time: 6 hours

Servings: 6

Ingredients:

6 white fish fillets, preferably fresh

2 tablespoons chopped parsley

2 tablespoons chopped basil

1 pinch turmeric

1 tablespoon lemon zest

2 tablespoons lemon juice

1 cup water or vegetable stock

Salt and pepper to taste

Directions:

1. In a bowl, mix the parsley with the basil, turmeric, lemon zest and lemon juice, as well as salt and freshly ground pepper.

2. Place the fish fillets in your crockpot and spread the herb mixture over each of them.

3. Carefully pour the water into the pot then cover and cook on low settings for 6 hours.

4. Serve the fish warm and fresh.

Nutritional information per serving

Calories: 105

Fat: 1.6g

Protein: 17.8g

Carbohydrates: 1.75g

Tips for making your own recipes

You can become your own best chef too! How do you make something you desire so much at the store as a treat, make it tasty but also healthy at the same time? First look at each ingredient that is on the list and secondly find out how to replace that ingredient with one that's good for you.

Let's take chocolate that you see on the shelves for an example. Usually chocolate would contain sugar to make it sweet. You'll see in some of the recipes I called for raw honey. You already know that this is a good replacement for sugar. Chocolate is actually derived from cocoa beans. You can buy cocoa beans grounded or you can ground them yourself but you'd have to add things like cocoa nibs, carob powder to make the chocolate not 100% dark and bitter. Add coconut oil and you've got yourself a delicious filling and sweet chocolate that is good for you! Want a crunch? Add your favorite nuts! Freeze it to make it into a block chocolate you see in the store.

Want an even more easier way to make your own chocolate? Buy chocolate (cocoa) butter that has no ingredients in it, add honey to make it sweet, add some nuts, and freeze it. You're done! No cooking required and prep time is 2 minutes.

You can find healthy replacements for whatever food you want to eat by making it yourself and researching good ingredients to replace the bad ones with. So go out there and try it out! Get creative and just maybe you'll teach Gordan Ramsey a thing or two. Or he might yell that your cooking is horrible and your hair looks bad. I'd still come over and eat though and ask for seconds so cheer up! Also, your hair looks good.

CHAPTER SEVEN: ALL GOOD THINGS MUST COME TO AN END BUT ALL BRILLIANT THINGS MUST CONTINUE

Congratulations! You journeyed through the book and made it to the end and that's no small feat! Usually people would buy a book and think just because they threw money at something that they'd solve their problem. If you made it this far and read the whole book, you now have a better understanding with how to lose fat and hopefully you've started doing the habits by now and started to write things down. You are one of the action takers, a doer. So I applaud your commitment to get through this book and deciding to better yourself.

So where to from here?

Keep taking action. Keep committed and be persistent. There will be many challenges you'll face on your journey to get the body you want, but when you do improve and when you finally get there, you'll know that you have earned it.

If you ever need any help, want extra free information, as a thank you for entrusting me and purchasing this book, feel free to contact me at my website and ask anything by simply subscribing! You are my billboard for my methods but also I really just want you to succeed and go beyond whatever fitness and health goal you initially set when you first started taking action from this book. To subscribe for free info the website is HTTP://www.paindoesnthurt.com

So now it's time to get in there and do it! Here's to your success!

Ceps Weston Domingo

ABOUT THE AUTHOR

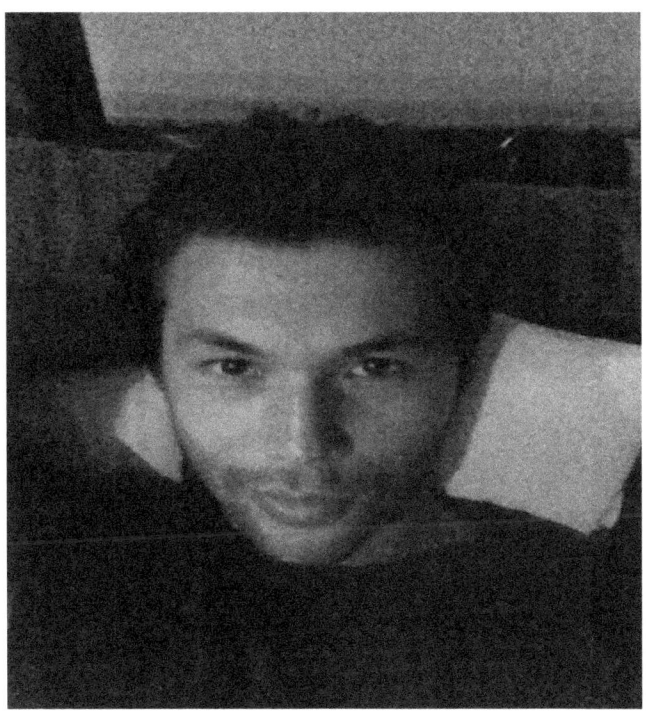

Ceps Weston Domingo is a personal trainer and nutritionist who is a mad scientist chef in the kitchen in his spare time. He has a blog for fitness, nutrition, business, recipes and succeeding in all aspects in life called HTTP://www. Paindoesnthurt.com On the website you can find out more about him, his advice and other best selling books such as: **30 day Paleo diet slow cooker recipe cookbook: Delicious, easy recipes to cook and eat at home that restore health and lose weight.** Ceps is dedicated to helping many people to all walks of life to achieve a healthy and happy lifestyle. It is his books and successes he dedicates to all the people who need help and to his mother.

Special thanks

Thanks to my good friends Delia, Owen, Sofia and Will for putting up with me and helping me out with my laptop when it broke in the midst of writing this book whilst yelling profanities at the screen.

Thanks to my Mom for everything. Without her nothing would be possible and you sure as heck wouldn't have seen this book! You're the strongest person I ever knew.

Finally thanks to all of you who purchased this book and trusting me. You guys rock!

If you like the book please leave a 5 star review! Thanks for purchasing!

References

1. Lim, S., Kim, K.M., Kim, M.J., Woo, S.J., Choi, H.S., Park, K.S., Jang, H.C., Meigs, J.B., & Wexler, D.J. (2013). The Association of maximum body weight on the development of Type 2 Diabetes and Microvascular Complications: MAXWEL Study doi: 10.1371/journal.pone.0080525.

2. Louzada, M.L., Rauber, F., Campagnolo, P.D, Vitolo, M.R. (2012). Sleep Duration and body mass index among southern Brazilian preschoolers.

3. De, J.L., Zhao, X., Mattingly, M.S., Zuber, S.M., Piaggi, P., Csako, G., Cizza, G. (2012). Poor sleep quality and sleep apnea are associated with higher resting energy expenditure in obese individuals with short sleep duration. NIDDIK Sleep extension study group.

4. Rosengren, A., Hauptman, P.J., Lappas, G., Olsson, L., Wilhelmsen, L., Swedberg, K. (2009). Big men and atrial fibrillation: effects of body size and weight gain on risk of atrial fibrillation in men.

5. Huang, P.H., Chen, Y.H., Tsai, H.Y., Chen, J.S., Wu, T.C., Lin, F.Y., Sata, M., Chen, J.W., Lin, S.J. (2010). Intake of red wine increases the number and functional capacity of circulating endothelial progenitor cells by enhancing nitric oxide bioavailability.

6.Chiva-Blanch, G., Urpi-sarda, M., Ros, E., Arranz, S., Valderas-Martinez, P., Casas, R., Sacanella, E., Llorach, R., Lamuela-Raventos, R.M., Andres-Lacueva, C., Estruch, R. Dealcoholized red wine decreases systolic and diastolic blood pressure and increases plasma nitric oxide: Short communication.

7.He, J., Ogden, L.G., Bazzano, L.A., Vupputuri, S., Loria, C., Whelton, P.K. (2002). Dietary sodium intake and incidence of congestive heart failure in overweight US men and women: first National Health and Nutrition Examination Survey Epidemiological Follow-up Study.

8.Hummel, S.L., Symour E.M., Brook, R.D., Kolias, T.J., Sheth, S.S., Rosenblum, H.R., Wells, J.M., Weder, A.B. (2012). Low-sodium dietary approaches to stop hypertension diet reduces blood pressure, arterial stiffness, and oxidative stress in hypertensive heart failure with preserved ejection fraction.

9.Akers, J.D., Cornett, R.A., Savla, J.S., Davy, K.P., Davy, B.M. (2012). Daily self-monitoring of body weight, step count, fruit/vegetable intake, and water consumption: a feasible and effective long-term weight loss maintenance approach.

158

10. Imai, S., Matsuda, M., Hasegawa, G., Fukui, M., Obayashi, H., Ozasa, N., Kajiyama, S. (2011). A simple meal plan of 'eating vegetables before carbohydrate' was more effective for achieving glycemic control than an exchange-based meal plan in Japanese patients with type 2 Diabetes.

11. Buijisse, B., Feskens, E.J., Schulze, M.B., Forouhi, N.G., Wareham, N.J., Sharp, S., Palli, D., Tognon, G., Halkjaer, J., Tjonneland, A., Jakobsen, M.U., Overad, K., van der, A. D.L., Du, Hu., Sorensen, T.I., Boeing, H. (2009). Fruit and vegetable intakes and subsequent changes in body weight in European population: results from the project on Diet, Obesity, and Genes (DiOgenes).

12. Giaconi, J.A., Yu, F., Stone, K.L., Pedula, K.L., Ensrud, K.E., Cauley, J.A., Hochberg, M.C., Coleman A.L., Study of Osteoporotic Fractures Research group. (2012). The association of consumption of fruits/Vegetables with decreased risk of glaucoma among older African-American women in the study of osteoportic fractures.

13. Riechman, S.E., Andrews, R.D., Maclean, D.A., Sheather, S. (2007). Statins and dietary and serum cholesterol are associated with increased lean mass following resistance training. Journals of Gerontology: Series A.

14. Marina, A.M., Man, Y.B., Nazimah, S.A., Amin, I. (2009). Antioxidant capacity and phenolic acids of virgin coconut oil.

15. Geliebter, A., Torbay, N., Bracco, E.F., Hashim, S.A., Van Itallie, T.B. (1983). Overfeeding with medium-chain triglyceride diet results in diminished deposition of fat.

16. Gupta, A., Malav, A., Singh, A., Gupta, M.K., Khinchi, M.P., Sharma, N., Agrawal, D. (2010). Coconut oil: The healthiest oil on earth. International journal of pharmaceutical sciences and research.

17. Munsters, M.J.M., Saris, W.H.M. (2012). Effects of meal frequency on metabolic profiles and substrate partitioning in lean healthy males

18. Campbell, S.C., Khalil, D.A., Payton, M.E., Arjmandi, B.H. (2010). One year-soy protein supplementation does not improve lipid profile in postmenopausal women.

19. Alekel, D.L., Van Loan, M.D., Koehler, K.J., Hanson, L.N., Stewart, J.W., Hanson, K.B., Kurzer, M.S., Peterson, C.T. (2010). The soy ioflavone for reducing bone loss (SIRBL study: a 3-y randomized controlled trial in postmenopausal women.

20. Adlecreutz, H., Hockerstedt, K., Bannwart, C., Bloigu, S., Hamalainen, E., Fotsis, T., Ollus, A. (1987). Effect of dietary components, including lignans and phytoestrogens on enterohepatic circulation and liver metabolism of estrogens and on sex hormone binding globulin (SHBG).

21. Siepmann, T., Roofeh, J., Kiefer, F.W., Edelson, D.G. (2011). Hypogandadism and erectile dysfunction associated with soy product consumption.

22. Xiong, J.S., Branigan, D., Li, M. (2009). Deciphering the MSG controversy.

23. Schwartz, G.R. (1999). Aspartame and breast and other cancers

24. Mortelmans, L.J., Van Loo, M., De Cauwer, H.G., Merlevede, K. (2008). Seizures and hypnatremia after excessive intake of diet coke.

25. Lenoir, M., Serre, F., Cantin, L., Ahmed, S.H. (2007). Intense Sweetness Surpasses Cocaine reward.

26. International Agency for Research on Cancer. Working Group on the Evaluation of
    Carcinogenic Risks to Humans, *Ingested Nitrates and Nitrites, and Cyanobacterial*
    Peptide Toxins IARC monographs on the evaluation of carcinogenic risks to humans ;.
    Vol. 94. 2007, Lyon: International Agency for Research on Cancer

27. Daxenberger, A., Breier, B.H., Sauerwein, H. (1998). Increased milk levels of insulin-like growth factor 1 (IGF-1) for the identification of bovine somatotropin (bST) treated cows.

28. Deangelo, A.B., George, M.H., Kilburn, S.R., Moore, T.M., and wolf, D.C. (1998). Carcinogenicity of Potassium Bromate Administered in the drinking water to Male. DOI: 10.1177/019262339802600501.

29. Stasiak, M., Lewinski, A., Karbownik-Lewinska, M. (2012). [Relationship between toxic effects of potassium bromate and endocrine glands].

30. Bray, G.A., Nielsen, S.J., and Popkin, B.M. (2004). Consumption of high-fructose corn syrup in beverages may play a role in the epidemic of obesity 1,2.

31. Biesiekierski, J.R., Newnham, E.D., Irving, P.M., Barret, J.S., Haines, M., Doecke, J.D., Shepherd, S.J., Muir, J.G., Gibson, P.R. (2011). Gluten causes gastrointestinal symptoms in subjects without celiac disease: a double-blind randomized placebo-controlled trial.

32. Chagas, C.E., Rogero, M.M., Martini, L.A. (2012). Evaluating the links between intake of milk/diary products and cancer.

33. Kokavec, A. (2008). Is decreased appetite for food a physiological consequence of alcohol consumption?

34. Arima, H., Kiyohara, Y., Kato, I., Tanizaki, Y., Kubo, M., Iwamoto, H., Tanaka, K., Abe, I., Fujishima, M. (2002). Alcohol reduces insulin-hypertension relationship in a general population: the Hisayama study.

35. Vingren, J.L., Hill, D.W., Buddhadev, H., Duplanty, A. (2013). Post resistance exercise ethanol ingestion and acute testosterone bioavailability.

36. Suter, P.M., Jequier, E., Schutz, Y. (1994). Effect of ethanol on energy expenditure.

162

37. Sierksma, A., Sarkola, T., Eriksson, C.J., van der Gaag, M.S., Grobbee, D.E., Hendriks, H.F. (2004). Effect of moderate alcohol consumption on plasma dehydropiandrosterone sulfate, testosterone, and estradiol levels in middle-aged men and postmenopausal women: a diet-controlled intervention study.

38. Valimaki, M., Tuominen, J.A., Huhtaniemi, I., Ylikahri, R. (1990). The pulsatile secretion of gonadotropins and growth hormone, and the biological activity of luteinizing hormone in men acutely intoxicated with ethanol.

39. Heikkonen, E., Ylikahri, R., Roine, R., Valimaki, M, Harkonen M., Salaspuro, M. (1996). The combined effect of alcohol and physical exercise on serum testosterone, luteinizing hormone, and corisol in males.

40. Koziris, L.P., Kraemer, W.J., Gordon, S.E., Incledon, T., Knuttgen, H.G. (1985). Effect of acute postexercise ethanol intoxication on the neuroendocrine response to resistance exercise.

41. Freed, D.L.J. (1999). Do dietary lecithins cause disease?

42. Pins, J.J., Geleva, D., Keenan, J.M., Frazel, C., O'connor, P.J., Cherney, L.M. (2002). Do whole-grain oat cereals reduce the need for antihypertensive medications and improve blood pressure control?

43. Hipkiss, A.R. (1998). Carnosine, a protective, anti-ageing peptide?

163

44. Rae, C., Digney, A.L., McEwan, S.R., Bates, T.C. (2003). Oral creatine monohydrate supplementation improves brain performance: a double blind, placebo-controlled, cross-over trail.

45. HTTP://en.wikipedia.org/wiki/Ketogenic_diet_%28Epilepsy%29

46. *Boden G, Sargrad K, Homko C, Mozzoli M, Stein TP. Effect of a low-carbohydrate diet on appetite, blood glucose levels, and insulin resistance in obese patients with type 2 diabetes. Ann Intern Med 2005;142:403–11.*

47. *Dashti, H.M., Mathew, T.C., Hussein, T., Asfar, S.K., Behbahani, A., Khoursheed, M.A., Al-Sayer, H.M., Bo-Abbas, Y.Y., Al-Zaid, N.S. (2004). Long-term effects of a ketogenic diet in obese patients.*

48. *O'connor, S.E., Richardson, C., Trescher, W.H., Byler, D.L., Sather, J.D., Micheal, E.H., Urbanik, K.B., Richards, J.L., Davis, R., Zupanc, M.L., Zupec-Kania, B. (2014). The ketogenic diet for the treatment of pediatric status epilepticus.*

49. *Azzam, R., Azar, N.J. (2013). Marked Seizure Reduction after MCT Supplementation.*

50. *Paoli, A., Bianco, A., Grimaldi, K.A., Lodi, A., Bosco, G. (2013). Long term successful weight loss with a combination biphasic ketogenic Mediterranean diet and Mediterranean diet maintenance protocol.*

51. *Soliman, A.T., Yasin, M., Kassem, A. (2012). Leptin in pediatrics: A hormone from adipocyte that wheels several functions in children.*

52. *Matsumoto, T., Miyawaki, C., Ue, H., Kanda, T., Yoshitake, Y., Moritani, T. (2001). Comparison of thermogenic sympathetic response to food intake between obese and non-obese young women.*

53. *Dirlewanger, M., di Vetta, V., Guenat, E., Battilana, P., Seematter, G., Schneiter, P., Jequier, E., Tappy, L. Effects of short-term carbohydrate or fat overfeeding on energy expenditure and plasma leptin concentrations in healthy female subjects.*

54. *Fried, S.K., Ricci, M.R., Russell, C.D., Laferrere, B. (2000). Regulation of leptin production in humans. J Nutr. Dec;130(12):3127S-3131S*

55. *Sofer, S., Eliraz, A., Kaplan, S., Voet, H., Fink, G., Kima, T., Madar, Z. (2011). Greater weight loss and hormonal changes after 6 months diet with carbohydrates eaten mostly at dinner.*

56. *Katayose, Y., Tasaki, M., Ogata, H., Nakata, Y., Tokuyama, K., Satoh, M. (2009). Metabolic rate and fuel utilization during sleep assessed by whole-body indirect calorimetry. Metabolism. 58(7):920-6.*

57. *Mischler, I., Vermorel, M., Montaurier, C., Mounier, R., Pialoux, V., Pequignot, J.M., Cottet-Emard, J.M., Coudert, J., Fellmann, N. (August 2003). Prolonged daytime exercise repeated over 4 days increases sleeping heart rate and metabolic rate. Can J Appl Physiol.*